INSANE TRAINING

ST. MARTIN'S GRIFFIN ❧ NEW YORK

GARAGE TRAINING, POWERLIFTING, BODYBUILDING, AND ALL-OUT BAD-ASS WORKOUTS

INSANE TRAINING

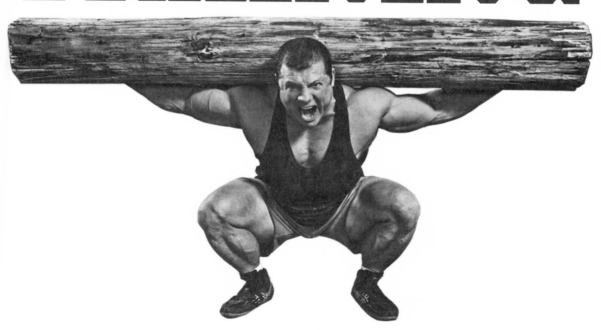

MATT KROCZALESKI

www.stmartins.com

Designed by Anna Gorovoy

The Library of Congress Cataloging-in-Publication Data is available upon request.

ISBN 978-1-250-02986-7 (trade paperback)
ISBN 978-1-250-02987-4 (e-book)

St. Martin's Griffin books may be purchased for educational, business, or promotional use. For information on bulk purchases, please contact Macmillan Corporate and Premium Sales Department at 1-800-221-7945, extension 5442, or write specialmarkets@macmillan.com.

First Edition: October 2014

10 9 8 7 6 5 4 3 2 1

I would like to dedicate this book to my three sons, Logan, Garrett, and Maxx. It is my hope that in leading by example I will continue to teach and inspire you to achieve all of your dreams and goals in life. The bond of unconditional love that we share means more to me than you boys will ever know. Thank you for being such amazing sons. As a father, I could not be more proud of the young men you boys have become.

CONTENTS

CONTENTS

INSANE
TRAINING

INTRODUCTION

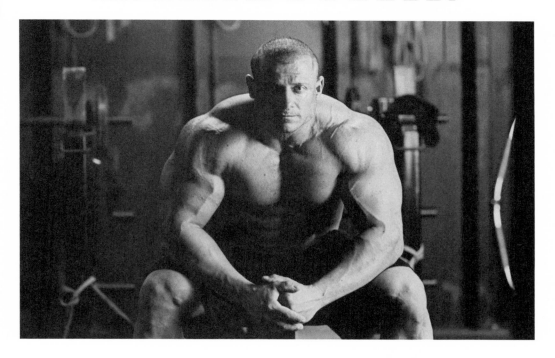

For those of you who have never heard of me, my name is Matthew Kroczaleski, but in the lifting world I'm better known as Matt Kroc or simply Kroc. I was born with an innate desire—a need, even—to build enormous muscles and freakish strength. That need has been there as long as I can remember. When I was five years old I recall seeing a large muscular guy and thinking, "Wow, that's how I want to be!" I started training consistently with weights by age nine, having made my first weight set out of empty milk jugs filled with sand. I placed them on a bent bar that I found in the woods and made my first weight bench from a six-foot-long two-by-twelve lying across two cinder blocks. I was immediately hooked, and those first days in my backyard deep in the woods evolved into a passion that has never subsided. Even though I started young and educated myself early, my success did not come easily. I was genetically more suited for running than lifting, but I was passionate about strength and refused to listen to anyone who told me that my dreams were impossible. Over the years, there were many detractors, including coaches, peers, and even family members. I was determined and worked hard, but by the time I was a high school freshman, I was still only a paltry 118 pounds. I took solace in the belief that if I was willing to work hard enough and make the necessary sacrifices, then with time I could achieve anything I put my mind to. From the start, my true strength was not in my muscles but rather in my constant willingness to push myself farther and suffer more than anyone I've ever met.

By the time I graduated high school, I had built myself into a lean muscular 180 pounds, and then I left my small rural hometown to join the Marine Corps. Through a lengthy screening process and rigorous testing, I was fortunate enough to be selected for presidential security duty. My tour of duty included time in Washington, D.C., where I provided security for the homes of admirals and generals assigned to the Pentagon as well as some of the Joint Chiefs of Staff. I was also chosen to be part of a security team for the then secretary of state Warren Christopher at the United Nations conferences in New York City. Later, I would be assigned to Marine Security Company at the presidential retreat Camp David during President Clinton's time in office. Throughout my time in the Marines, I continued to train extremely hard and often went to great lengths to ensure that I was able to get all of the necessary training in.

After leaving the Marines, I entered college. Six years later, I exited as a licensed pharmacist. I started college as a bachelor, but by the time I graduated, I was married and had three amazing sons, my youngest being born several months before I graduated. Even though I went to pharmacy school full-time and worked enough hours to support my wife and children, I still always made time to train with intensity sufficient to attain my goals. In pharmacy school, I would often be in classes all day and then work until closing time at a pharmacy that was nearly an hour away. I returned home to eat and finally drag myself down to the gym in the middle of the night to train. I was exhausted and wanted nothing more than to climb into bed, but I knew that there was no other option if I wished to achieve my goals. I had to literally break into the building that held the school's private weight-lifting club since it was locked up tight by the time I arrived. The gym was housed in the basement of the oldest building on campus. The walls were covered in hand-painted murals, hot water pipes traversed the ceiling, and much of the equipment was handmade by the original members of the club back in the '70s. It was the perfect environment to torture myself, and I loved training there. This was the scenario when I was training for my first national powerlifting championship. Down there in the middle of the night, I would stare into the mirror and have conversations with myself. I would question my own resolve and challenge myself to prove that I was willing to give everything. Some of the best training sessions of my life occurred during that time, alone in the hot, dark dungeonlike gym. Sweat poured, blood flowed, and I grew stronger physically and mentally. I went on to place third in my weight class that year, standing on a national-championship podium for the first time. It would be another six years before I ascended to the top of the podium at the WPO, World Powerlifting Organization, world championships, and it did not come easily.

In the years between those defining moments, I battled testicular cancer and underwent several surgeries to repair torn tendons that I ruptured in training. From the beginning, adversity was never a stranger to me. Every obstacle I successfully negotiated strengthened my belief that nothing could stop me. During nearly two decades of competitive powerlifting, I suffered numerous injuries, including muscle and tendon tears, separated joints, and torn ligaments. I never once doubted my ability to come back stronger—even when many others did. I was written off by many critics on more than one occasion, but nothing motivated me more than the opportunity to silence them. I considered injuries simply bumps in the road on my way to achieving my goals. I continued to doggedly chase my ultimate goal for several years, and then in 2009 I finally achieved it, attaining the highest powerlifting total ever recorded in the 220-pound class by squatting 1,003 pounds, bench-pressing 738 pounds, and deadlifting 810 pounds, for a combined 2,551 pounds. In this book, I will explain how I trained, recount the many things I endured, and show you detailed examples of the exact training programs I used to obtain my success.

ONE
CRAZY KID

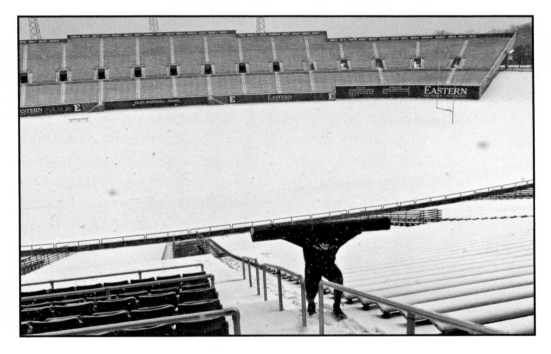

My insanity toward training was with me from the time I was a young child. By the time I was in third grade, I was training for our school's annual track and field day. It was the most important day of the year to me, and I dreamed about winning three blue ribbons all year long in anticipation of it. The standing long jump, fifty-yard dash, and softball throw were my own personal Olympics, and I desired nothing less than gold in all three. At nine years old, I really didn't know much about training, but I knew that I wanted to win and, instinctively, that working hard was the best way to achieve my goal. I would go out and run timed half miles and do endless sprints up the sand hill behind our mobile home. After reading about Herschel Walker in *Sports Illustrated,* I added push-ups, sit-ups, and chin-ups to my training regimen. My mother would constantly worry that I was somehow doing too much and that I would injure myself, but I didn't let that discourage me from my training. Years later in high school, those sand-hill sprints would include a log on my back, and I remember friends coming over and waiting for me to finish my "log hills," as I called them, so we could go out.

As a child, I would often turn anything I could into part of my training. My brother and I would ride our Huffy BMX bikes to baseball practice. The ride was several miles down country dirt roads and had a number of hills along the way. Several of these hills were relatively steep and fairly long, and most kids would immediately hop off of their bikes and push them up the hill. I, on other hand, refused to do this and felt as if dismounting my bike was akin to surrendering in a war against the hill. No matter how bad my legs and lungs burned, I would continue to slowly pump my legs up and down until I reached the summit of each hill. I always abhorred losing, even if it was against something as inanimate as those hills.

TWO
THE BENCH PRESS

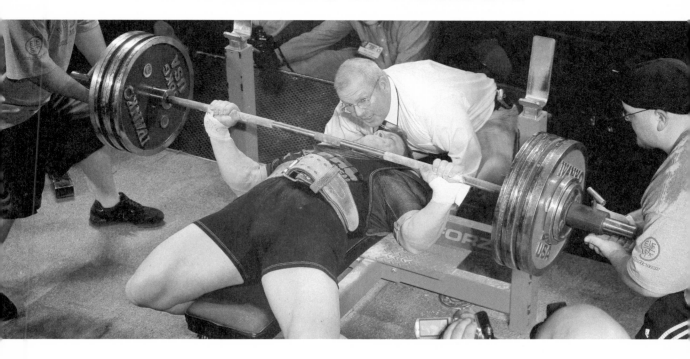

There is no denying that the bench press is the king of upper-body exercises. It is a matter of pride in the gym, as well as the most common measure of one's weight-lifting acumen. We all want to bench big, and most of us probably enjoy performing this exercise more than any other. And, of course, if performed correctly, the bench press will give us results that match our enthusiasm for it by adding slabs of beef to our pecs, shoulders, and triceps.

So if this is all true, why do so many people still possess tiny bird chests and a bench max that looks like an IQ score? Simply lying down on the bench and heaving the weight around isn't enough; it is performing the bench press correctly that makes all the difference. I'm referring not only to the correct use of form but also proper weight selection, intelligent programming, appropriate assistance exercises, and knowledge of how changes in technique affect both the primary muscles used and the amount of weight that can be moved.

FORM AND TECHNIQUE

First, let's talk about the proper setup for benching, since this is both literally and figuratively where we begin. Your setup and technique will depend on your primary goals. I will cover both how to set up optimally for moving the most weight possible and what changes to make when your goal is to build the biggest chest possible. The primary difference between the two is the lower back arch and the degree to which you employ it. Powerlifters will want to maximize their arch, which will not only decrease the range of motion but also effectively increase leverage, allowing you to move more weight. Bodybuilders will want less of an arch so that the muscle is worked through a greater range of motion.

SETUP AND FOOT PLACEMENT

I will first cover the powerlifting-type setup, since this is the more complex of the two. First, lie down on the bench and grab the bar with an underhand grip. Slide backward along the bench and under the bar until your upper ab area is directly under the bar. Now, while staying in this position, tuck your feet back under the bench, directly beneath your hips and with the balls of your feet in contact with the floor and your heels raised. While keeping your feet in the same place, slide your body back toward the bottom of the bench until your torso is in the proper position to bench. At this point, your lower back should be arched quite high. Ensure your hips are in contact with the bench, and then dig your traps and upper shoulder blades (which should be pulled back together as much as possible) into the bench. Pinching your shoulder blades back and together not only provides stability under heavy weights but also helps decrease the range of motion since it pushes your chest up and pulls your shoulders back. Maintain this position while you adjust your grip, unrack the bar, and perform your bench press.

Bodybuilders will still want to set your feet first, but they can either be placed underneath your hips, as in the description above, or with the entire foot flat on the floor out in front of you. If you have difficulty keeping your hips on the bench while pressing, I would suggest trying the style with your feet underneath you since this form still allows you to use a good degree of leg drive but is more conducive to keeping your hips on the bench while doing so. Then simply lie back and dig your traps into the bench for stability: there is no need for a big arch since you do not want to decrease the range of motion.

LEG DRIVE

Many lifters are confused about exactly what leg drive is and even more so about how to effectively use it. Fortunately, it is really quite simple. With either foot placement described above, keep your feet planted firmly against the floor and maintain a moderate amount of tension in your legs as you bring the bar to your chest. As the bar touches your chest and you begin to reverse direction, push hard with your legs as you drive the bar off your chest. This will help to pop the bar off your chest, and the added momentum will assist you in getting the bar through your sticking point and all the way to lockout.

BAR PATH

The correct bar path is another facet of the bench press that many lifters do not understand. The most mechanically efficient bar path is a gradual arc from just below your nipple line at the bottom of the movement to roughly above the base of your neck at lockout. The exact points will vary slightly depending on your individual leverages. This groove will allow you to bench the greatest weight possible. To perform this properly, tuck your elbows in toward your sides as you lower the bar, aiming for a point just below your nipple line when the bar is touching your chest. The lowering of the bar must be performed in the correct groove because your body will naturally want to follow that same path as you press upward. The concentric and eccentric portions of the bench press should appear as mirror images of each other. As you begin to drive the bar from your chest, continue to keep your elbows tucked. As the bar approaches the midpoint of the movement, however, gradually begin rotating your elbows out until they are fully flared at lockout. This should always be performed carefully since flaring too fast or too much too soon will send the bar back over your head and into the racks and can put a lot of stress on the shoulder joint if done excessively. This technique can also be effectively employed when you hit your sticking point on a difficult lift, since the flaring allows you to straighten your arms to a small degree without the bar actually having to move upward.

ELBOW POSITION

Tucking your elbows in at the bottom of the movement decreases shoulder rotation, thereby taking stress off the shoulder joint, and it also takes pressure off the pec tendon, decreasing the chance of a pec tear. This position thus allows you to lift more weight by improving your leverage. When the bar is at your chest, your elbows, wrists, and the bar should all be in a perfectly straight vertical line when viewed from the side. Do not allow the wrists to bend backward with the bar being held back behind the arm. Not only does this place a lot of stress on your wrist, it can negatively affect your leverage. Big benchers have actually suffered broken arms by using this technique.

GRIP

Generally speaking, there are three different ways to grip the bar: with a full grip (thumb wrapped all the way around the bar), with a false, or thumbless, grip, in which the thumb is held behind the bar; and with the thumb held straight out along the bar. Regardless of which grip you use, you should always attempt to squeeze the bar as hard as possible and push out to the sides as if trying to pull the bar apart. This will increase your ability to engage your triceps and allow you to bench more weight.

While most lifters realize that using a wider grip will focus more on the chest and that a close grip hits the triceps hard, few realize that not only where but also how you grip the bar affects muscle recruitment. Selecting the appropriate grip is critical to ensuring you are working with and not against your own strengths and leverages. Changing the position of your thumb affects the position of your elbows. The full grip rotates your hand outward to a greater degree, thus rotating your elbows out and using the chest to the greatest degree of the three grips. With the thumbless grip, the hands are turned in more toward the body, making it easier to tuck the elbows on the descent and recruiting the triceps to a greater degree. Gripping the bar with the thumb along the bar is a compromise of the two. So a lifter with a comparatively stronger chest (or one looking to work the chest to the highest degree possible) would benefit most by using a wide full grip, whereas a lifter with extremely strong triceps would be able to lift the most weight with a relatively narrow thumbless grip.

ASSISTANCE EXERCISES

Assistance exercises are properly determined by the lifter's strengths and weaknesses. Maintaining balance among your muscle groups is not only vital to preventing injury but also allows you to lift the most weight. Identifying your weaknesses in the bench is relatively easy, assuming the problem is not technique related. Difficulty locking out the weight at the top of the movement is nearly always due to a relative weakness in the triceps, whereas having difficulty getting the weight moving at the bottom of the movement is typically related to a weak chest. However, if the bar is barely leaving the chest or isn't moving from it at all, that can sometimes be attributed to a lat weakness, again assuming the problem is not form or ego related: if you're unracking the bar and it's stapling you to the bench, odds are that you just aren't being realistic as far as your true strength levels are concerned.

STRENGTHENING YOUR LOCKOUT

REVERSE BAND PRESSES

The exercise I prefer most for fixing a lockout weakness is reverse band presses. The reasons for this are several. Even though the exercise focuses on your lockout, it still allows you to work through a full range of motion and to press the bar in your normal groove. It also teaches you to push the bar from your chest explosively, because if you fail to do this, the momentum from the bands will be lost and locking the weight out will be extremely difficult. To set this exercise up, simply loop a pair of the strong bands around the top of a power cage (one on either side) and then hook them around the ends of the bar where you would normally place the collars. Place a dumbbell bench inside the rack, and you're all set to bench. This setup will typically take approximately 150 pounds off the bar when it is at your chest and next to nothing at lockout, depending on the height of the cage, the bench height, and your arm length.

BOARD PRESSES

Board presses are another very effective tool for fixing your lockout. Depending on your arm length and where specifically the bar stalls when you're pressing, you will use boards two and five inches thick when performing this exercise. Typically the "boards" are constructed from two-by-six pine boards and are usually nailed, screwed, or glued together to achieve the desired thickness. I have found that making the pressing area about eighteen inches long and having a six-inch handle works quite well. To perform this exercise, you simply have a partner hold the boards on your chest while you're benching. If you don't have someone available to do that, I have found that the boards can be easily held in place by securing them to your chest with a single knee wrap tied around you.

STRENGTHENING THE BOTTOM PORTION OF THE PRESS

Technique issues aside, the ability to drive the bar off your chest largely comes from your pectoral muscles and lats. Here, I focus on strengthening the pecs. Any exercise that allows you to work through a greater range of motion will typically help improve the "pop" off your chest. Dumbbell benching and the use of a cambered bar are the methods I prefer most when addressing a relatively weak chest. Dumbbell benching prevents you from bouncing the bar off your chest and also allows you to work through a greater range of motion by allowing you to get a deeper stretch at the bottom of the movement.

The cambered bar is also sometimes referred to as the MacDonald bar, in honor of the legendary bencher Mike MacDonald, who often used this bar in his training. MacDonald once held every bench-press world record from the 181-pound class all the way up to 242 pounds.

The bar has a two-inch camber to it, allowing the lifter to lower the bar two inches farther than with a standard bar. One important thing to note here is that you must be very careful when first using the MacDonald bar because injury can easily result from the increased range of motion. Also expect the amount of weight you can use with the MacDonald bar to initially be significantly less than your normal bench, especially if your primary weakness in the bench is the bottom of the lift.

PROGRAMMING

Effective programming for the bench press involves a well-planned progression in the amount of weight used, sufficiently addresses and prevents overtraining, stimulates hypertrophy, and reinforces proper technique. The following program is one that I frequently use with clients looking to add not only pounds to their bench press but some pec mass as well. With this program, it is not uncommon for me to see an increase of twenty to fifty pounds in a lifter's bench press over a sixteen-week training period.

The key to using this program effectively is starting with an accurate max. All too often, lifters overestimate their max or use a number they were previously capable of. It is essential to use your current true max that is obtained using proper form. Failure to do so will only result in overtraining and difficulty in progressing from week to week, negating the effectiveness of the program. In plain English: check your ego to make the most of this program. It is also important to note that the lifter's max is not to be recalculated at any point during the program. Strength increases have been factored into the design of this program, and adjusting the weights used during the program will decrease its effectiveness. This program is also designed for the athlete to bench only once every seven days. Attempting to train the bench more often than this when following this program will quickly lead to an overtrained state and a reduction in strength.

16-WEEK WEIGHT PROGRESSION

WEEK 1	5 x 10 x 60% (5 sets of 10 reps at 60% of 1 rep max)
WEEK 2	5 x 8 x 70%
WEEK 3	5 x 6 x 75%
WEEK 4	5 x 4 x 80%
WEEK 5	5 x 10 x 60%
WEEK 6	5 x 7 x 75%
WEEK 7	5 x 5 x 80%
WEEK 8	5 x 3 x 85%
WEEK 9	5 x 10 x 60%
WEEK 10	4 x 6 x 80%
WEEK 11	4 x 4 x 85%
WEEK 12	4 x 2 x 90%
WEEK 13	5 x 10 x 60%
WEEK 14	3 x 5 x 85%
WEEK 15	3 x 3 x 90%
WEEK 16	3 x 1 x 95%

THREE
DEADLIFTING

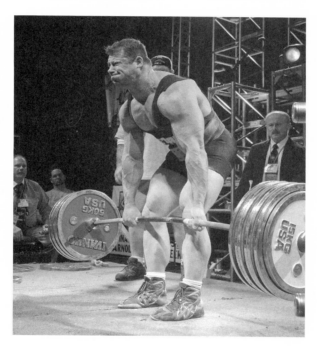

Deadlifting is the base upon which all real back strength is built. There is not a more raw or true-to-life exercise. You bend over and pick up something heavy—that's it. The deadlift's simplicity, however, is also the reason it is so effective. It stresses every major muscle group in your posterior chain, but none more so than your back. It works your back from the base of your erectors to the top of your traps. You can always spot a guy with a big deadlift. He possesses powerful yoked traps and a back thickness that you can't obtain any other way. Ronnie Coleman and Johnnie Jackson possess two of the thickest and most powerful-looking backs to ever appear on a bodybuilding stage. It's no coincidence that they are both capable of deadlifting more than eight hundred pounds.

Training the deadlift is also surprisingly simple. Hit it hard and heavy and then let your body rest and grow. Generally speaking, the rep schemes are going to be lower than most other compound movements. Sets of 5–10 repetitions generally work best for bodybuilding purposes, and for pure strength it is very common to work up to heavy triples, doubles, and even singles on a regular basis. There's also no need for fancy techniques like drop sets, supersets or rest-pause sets for deadlifts. While deadlifting isn't a highly complex movement, it is an incredibly taxing one. Thus, you have to be cautious not to over-train your back. This is especially true if you're also squatting heavy and working your back hard with lots of heavy rowing movements.

The deadlift can often be increased most effectively by working in short three-week waves followed by a down or deload week. Essentially, the weights are increased each week for a three-week period, often with a decrease in the rep range, then trained lightly or not at all the fourth week before entering the next wave with progressively heavier weights. I have had a lot of success with this style of programming for myself, training partners and clients that I work with. Another key facet of programming deadlift training is recognizing and preventing overtraining. As you get significantly stronger, your volume and training frequency will often need to be decreased. This is especially true with very strong powerlifters or strongmen. For those who are able to deadlift in excess of seven hundred pounds and prefer to train with heavy weights, I have often found that deadlifting every other week works quite well. The lower back is still trained hard on the in between weeks but with different exercises like good mornings, weighted back raises, reverse hypers, and pull-throughs. This allows the lifter to train consistently heavy, facilitating significant strength gains but also effectively mitigating the likeliness of overtraining. There are many other effective methods of programming the deadlift, but these are the ones that I have had the most success with.

Deadlifting is comprised of two main styles, or techniques, one being the sumo style, named thus because it resembles a sumo wrestler's stance, in which the feet are out wide and the hands are placed inside the legs. The other technique is the conventional style, where the stance is narrower, generally shoulder-width or closer, and the hands are placed outside the legs when gripping the bar. To generalize, we would say that smaller, thinner lifters tend to perform better with the sumo style and larger, thicker lifters tend to perform better with the conventional style due to the leverages involved. . However, there are certainly exceptions to the rule. For example, the many-times world champion Lamar Gant was able to deadlift over six hundred pounds at only 132-pound body weight using the conventional style. Vince Anello, weighing less than two hundred pounds, was another lifter who set world records in the deadlift using the conventional style, pulling in excess of eight hundred pounds at a body weight of 198. At the other end of the spectrum, O. D. Wilson was a mammoth super heavyweight that deadlifted close to nine hundred pounds using the sumo style. There are also other world-class lifters who were able to deadlift equally well with either style, including Chuck Vogelpohl, who deadlifted well over eight hundred pounds using both styles—he was even known to switch between the two styles on consecutive attempts in the same meet. So, as you can see, while we are able to make generalizations, it is really up to the individual lifter to figure out what style best suits his or her individual strengths, weaknesses, and leverages.

Sumo style is generally considered more technique and leverage driven than the conventional style, which is generally regarded as more about overall brute strength. When using the sumo style, the athlete's stance, setup, and technique must be perfect or the attempt will often fail. This isn't to say that technique is unimportant for the conventional style, just that it doesn't play as significant a role as it does in the sumo style. As with any lift, technique is always an important factor in moving the most amount of weight possible.

While both styles use many of the same muscle groups, the conventional style works the entire posterior chain, including your hamstrings, glutes, erectors, upper back musculature, and traps, whereas the sumo style tends to involve more of the hips and takes advantage of optimal leverages. If you're not a competitive powerlifter and are merely using deadlifting as a tool to increase the strength and size of your posterior chain musculature, then it would definitely be preferable to train using the conventional style. Conventional deadlifting will have a greater carryover to everyday movements outside the gym and will be more applicable to increasing performance in other athletic endeavors.

HAND PLACEMENT AND GRIP

The type of grip you use and your hand placement will essentially be the same whether you're pulling using a conventional or sumo style. With a few minor exceptions, the width of your hand placement on the bar is determined by your shoulder width. You will want to grip the bar with your arms hanging straight down from your shoulders. This allows you to use the maximum length of your arms, which shortens the range of motion and, in terms of leverage, puts you in an advantageous starting position. A grip that is too narrow or too wide will cause you to bend down farther, thus increasing the range of motion and negatively affecting your leverage in the starting position. One notable exception to this rule would be thickly built lifters with a large midsection. Many lifters with this build find it to be advantageous to grip the bar slightly outside shoulder width and open up their stance wide enough to allow their stomach to descend between their legs when they move into the starting position. This setup allows lifters with this build to keep the bar closer to their center of gravity throughout the lift, thus increasing their leverage and the amount of weight they're able to move.

Deadlifting is typically performed with an over-under grip, or what is sometimes referred to as a mixed grip. This simply means that one hand is in an overhand grip position and the other hand is holding the bar in an underhand grip position. This provides a stronger grip because it allows a lifter to hold on to larger weights than they would be able to otherwise since the bar is not able to roll in one direction out of the lifter's hands. Most people will find it beneficial to put their dominant hand in the underhand position because the underhand position is the more difficult of the two grips to maintain and typically the dominant hand of a person is the stronger one.

An alternative grip is the hook grip. It has been widely used by Olympic weightlifters, and recently powerlifters have taken notice. This grip has helped a number of lifters that lack the grip strength to hold on to heavy deadlifts when using the over-under grip. The other major benefit is that the hook grip takes some of the pressure off the distal-biceps tendon, by eliminating the need for an underhand grip. This can be helpful for a lifter coming back from surgery to repair a torn biceps tendon or for anyone wishing to reduce the risk of the injury beforehand.

The hook grip is performed by taking a double overhand grip on the bar while trapping one's thumbs within the grip. This is done by gripping the bar with the thumbs of both hands wrapped around the bar as far as possible and then placing the fingers over the top of the thumb, effectively trapping it against the bar. With this grip, the greater the amount of weight on the bar, the more pressure there is trapping the thumb within the grip. While this can be a very effective technique when used correctly, it also requires a higher degree of pain tolerance since the pressure on the thumb can become quite severe, especially when deadlifting very heavy weights. This technique is also a bit easier for people with larger hands to use because it is easier for them to wrap their thumb farther around the bar, which gives them more surface area to trap the thumb in their hand, providing a more stable grip. If you plan to use the hook grip, be sure to have patience with it. Many lifters will find it very painful at first but will often build tolerance to the discomfort over time. This grip is also not meant to be used for high rep sets (i.e., eight reps or more) and is best suited for singles, doubles, and possibly triples.

STARTING POSITION

While the most optimal starting position will be dictated by the individual lifter's leverages and body type, there are definitely some general rules that will apply to most lifters.

DISTANCE FROM THE BAR

While you will hear many coaches and trainers say that the closer you are to the bar, the better, this is not necessarily true in all cases. Some lifters who stand too close to the bar at the start will find that the bar will actually have to go forward as it passes the knees, thus making the lift longer and more difficult to complete.

The best way to determine a lifter's optimal starting position is to observe the lift from the side. If you do not have a trusted training partner, you can use a video camera for this. You want to watch the bar path as the bar leaves the floor and starts to ascend. When the bar leaves the floor, it should travel upward in a straight line. If it moves in toward the lifter as it leaves the floor, then the lifter is setting up too far away from the bar; conversely, if the bar moves away from the lifter, he or she is setting up too close to the bar. You also want to watch the position of the bar when a lifter sets it down after the completion of each rep during a multiple-rep set, since this is often the optimal place to begin the lift.

Since the starting position and technique are so different in the conventional and sumo styles, we will talk about the proper technique for each style separately.

CONVENTIONAL DEADLIFTING

The lifter's head should be up and in a neutral position, looking straight ahead. It is neither necessary nor desirable to look upward excessively because doing so can lead to a loss of balance. The lower back should not be excessively rounded or arched, instead a neutral spine position should be maintained throughout the lift. The hips should be down and back, which will leave the shins in an almost vertical position. You may hear some coaches advocate a high hip position at the start of a deadlift. There are some lifters for whom this works very well, but generally speaking those lifters are genetically gifted with a very short torso and long arms and legs, giving them perfect leverage for the deadlift. When lifters who are not built this way attempt to use this form, they often find themselves stiff legging the deadlift and locking out their knees too early, which results in their being in a poor position leverage wise and having a lot of difficulty finishing the lift. Lifters with extremely short torsos can also often get away with excessive rounding of the upper back during the lift. There have actually been a few world record holders who used this technique to their advantage. But, again, lifters not built in a way ideal for this technique will have difficulty getting their shoulders back at the top of the lift, and so it should be avoided.

When initiating the lift, lifters should engage their quads and attempt to push their feet straight down through the floor, and some lifters find it helpful to envision themselves actually pushing the floor away from the bar and describe the movement as a sort of leg press while holding the bar. At the beginning of the lift, it is important to move the bar away from the floor as fast and as explosively as possible since the momentum gained from this will aid greatly in completing the lift. This is why you often hear coaches at meets yelling, "Grip and rip!" as their lifters set up at the bar. This does not mean that the bar should be jerked from the floor; on the contrary, it is important to move the bar smoothly away from the floor to stay in the proper groove while initiating the lift. To avoid initiating the lift with a jerking motion, a lifter should take the slack out of the bar just before exploding upward. This is accomplished by pulling up on the bar only hard enough to make it bend a bit just before ripping the bar off the floor. This tension is only placed on the bar for a split second before initiating the lift to effectively ensure a smooth start to the lift without wasting any of the lifter's energy. When performed properly by an experienced lifter, it happens so quickly that it is almost indiscernible to the naked eye.

When getting ready to begin the lift, the lifter should be down at the bar for as short a time as humanly possible before initiating the pull. Of the three main powerlifts, the deadlift is the only one that begins without an eccentric phase of the lift happening first. This almost entirely negates a stretch reflex, which helps a lifter in most exercises begin the concentric phase. World record holder Fred Hatfield, also known as Dr. Squat, often leaped high into the air several times right before starting the deadlift in an attempt to establish the stretch reflex. The longer a lifter takes to set up at the beginning of the deadlift, the more difficult it becomes to initiate the lift explosively.

Once the bar reaches the knees, the lifter should be attempting to bring the hips forward and throw the shoulders back. During the entire lift, the lifter should attempt to keep the shoulders behind the bar. While this is technically not possible, envisioning this will help the lifter maintain the optimal upper-body position. As the bar nears lockout, the lifter should be attempting to push the hips through and pull the shoulders back, and the hips and knees should straighten simultaneously. If the knees lock out before the lift is complete, the bar will be out away from the body, the lifter will be in a poor position for leverage, and the lift will be difficult to finish.

SUMO DEADLIFTING

When setting up for a sumo deadlift, in most cases you will want to be as close to the bar as possible. This usually means the bar will be resting against your shins at the start of the lift since you want the bar to be as close to your center of gravity as possible. Your feet will be out wide and your toes will be pointing out. It is important that when you descend down to the bar, you do so in the same groove and with the same technique that you want the ascent to go up in. This is because your body will instinctively want to follow that same path. When you watch the very best sumo deadlifters in the world set up, you will notice that they descend to the bar to get in position with perfect form. If you just bend over and grab the bar with your butt up in the air, when you initiate the lift you will have to fight against your hips, which will want to shoot up and out—something you definitely don't want.

Once you're in the proper starting position and are ready to initiate the pull again, you want to take the slack out of the bar just before ripping the bar up, just as you would in the conventional style. When you start your pull, you want to force your knees out hard and push out sideways with your feet. This will help move your hips in toward the bar, giving you the best leverage possible. To help visualize this, picture the floor as if there is a large crack running straight between your legs from front to back. Your goal is to push the floor apart and make that crack wider. Again, pushing out in this manner will bring your hips in quickly toward the bar, putting you in the best leverage position to lift the most weight. You will want to keep your head up and your back flat and throw your shoulders back. The bar should stay in tight against your body throughout the pull and gently slide up against your legs the entire time. As with the conventional-style deadlift, your knees and hips should lock out simultaneously.

PROGRAMMING FOR THE DEADLIFT

Effective programming for the deadlift involves a well-planned progression in the amount of weight used, sufficiently addresses and prevents overtraining, stimulates hypertrophy, and reinforces proper technique. With this program, it is not uncommon to see an increase of twenty to fifty pounds in a lifter's deadlift over a sixteen-week training period, and I have witnessed as much as a ninety-pound increase. With this program, you only deadlift once per week—preferably three to four days after squatting. You will also notice that there is no deadlifting every fourth week. This is to allow sufficient recovery and prevent overtraining. Deadlifting is very taxing, and the lower back muscles are often stressed heavily when squatting and during other heavy back movements, so the break will be needed. During this week you can still train the lower back muscles but with different exercises like good mornings, weighted back raises, reverse hypers, and pull-throughs, and the rep ranges should be kept in the ten-to-twenty range.

The key to using this program effectively is starting with an accurate max. All too often, lifters overestimate their max or use a number they were previously capable of. It is essential to use your current true max that is obtained using proper form. Failure to do so will only result in overtraining and difficulty in progressing from week to week, negating the effectiveness of the program. In plain English: check your ego to make the most of this program. It is also important to note that the lifter's max is not to be recalculated at any point during the program. Strength increases have been factored into the design of this program, and adjusting the weights used during the program will decrease its effectiveness.

16-WEEK WEIGHT PROGRESSION

WEEK 1	(after warming up) 5 x 5 x 70% (5 sets of 5 reps at 70% of 1 rep max)
WEEK 2	5 x 3 x 75%
WEEK 3	5 x 1 x 80%
WEEK 4	no deadlifting, but you may work lower back with alternate exercises in the 10+ rep range
WEEK 5	5 x 5 x 75%
WEEK 6	5 x 3 x 80%
WEEK 7	5 x 1 x 85%
WEEK 8	no deadlifting
WEEK 9	4 x 5 x 80%
WEEK 10	4 x 3 x 85%
WEEK 11	4 x 1 x 90%
WEEK 12	no deadlifting
WEEK 13	3 x 5 x 85%
WEEK 14	3 x 3 x 90%
WEEK 15	3 x 1 x 95%
WEEK 16	no deadlifting
WEEK 17	retest your max

FOUR
SQUATTING

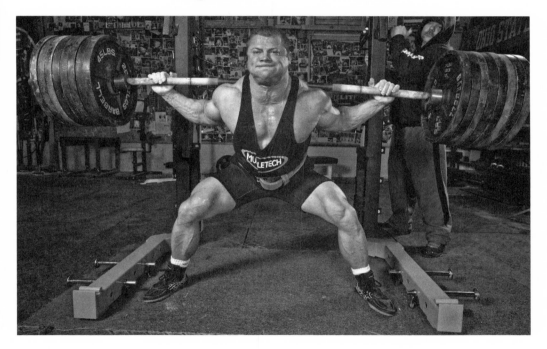

BAR POSITION

The first thing we're going to talk about is bar position. There's a lot more to where you hold the bar on your back than you might think. The position in which the bar is held on the lifter's back will play a role in determining the angle of forward lean of the lifter. The lower the bar is held on the lifter's back, the greater the angle of forward lean will be. Powerlifters often hold the bar in what is referred to as the low bar position, which is typically across the lower area of the rear deltoid muscles. There is a shelf for the bar created in that area when a lifter pulls his or her elbows back to grip the bar. The advantage of carrying the bar in this position is twofold. First, this is typically a more comfortable position to place the bar, especially with heavier weights. Second, and more important, the resulting forward lean provides many lifters with increased leverage to move heavier weights. The downside to this technique is that the increased forward lean of the upper torso causes the hips to remain higher during the descent and requires the lifter to squat deeper to reach parallel. In competitive powerlifting, parallel is defined as the depth a lifter reaches when the crease at the front of the hip joint at the top of the lifter's thigh is equal horizontally to the top of the knee. According to powerlifting rules, this plane must be broken for a competition squat to be considered a good lift.

The other position the bar is commonly held in is known as the high bar position. This technique is most frequently used by Olympic weightlifters. The bar is carried high on the top of the trapezius muscle and near the base of the neck. The advantage of holding the bar here is that it allows the lifter to stay more upright, which means that reaching parallel is easier since the hips are not rotated forward by excessive lean.

HAND PLACEMENT

Generally speaking, it is preferential to grasp the bar with the hands as close to the shoulders as possible since doing so creates a tighter upper back and provides more stability throughout the lift. However, many lifters and especially the larger, more muscular athletes may find it difficult to place the hands in close to the shoulders because of flexibility issues in the shoulder joint and the sheer size of the muscles in the shoulders, upper arms, and upper back. However, they should still attempt to bring their grip in as close as possible. It is also preferable to grasp the bar with the thumb encircling the bar, which provides a better grip on the bar and helps prevent it from moving or rolling down the lifter's back during the execution of the squat. But, again, gripping the bar with the thumb encircling the bar versus having the thumb over the bar requires greater flexibility. A lifter should experiment with grip types and widths to find what feels most stable. Once the grip is secure, the lifter should pull down on the bar, forcing the elbows down and in, which also aids in creating greater stability. This position should be maintained throughout the lift.

REMOVING THE BAR FROM THE RACK AND SETTING UP

When setting up under the bar, the first thing athletes should do is take the proper grip and ensure they are centered correctly on the bar before moving to get underneath it. Once underneath the bar, they should position their body directly under the bar so that, when they have the bar in the proper position on their back, they can simply stand straight up to remove the bar from the rack. This seems simple, but many lifters waste energy by attempting to remove the bar from the rack while standing too far away from the bar, essentially performing a good-morning-type exercise to unrack the bar. This not only wastes energy and requires more effort but also places a lot of strain on the lower back, often causing the lifter to be leaning too far forward once the bar has been removed from the rack. The lifter's head should be kept up and looking forward, and the chest should be kept up as well to prevent the upper back from rounding.

Once the bar is free from the rack, the minimum amount of steps should be taken to get into the proper stance to begin the squat. You will often see athletes walking the bar out several feet away from the racks and shuffling their feet back and forth numerous times to get into the proper stance to begin their squat. This is both a waste of valuable energy and completely unnecessary. No more than two to three steps need to be taken to get into the proper stance. If the lifter squats with a relatively narrow stance, then only two steps—back with one foot and then back with the other—are required. These steps only need to be large enough to clear the racks by several inches. If the lifter uses a wide-stance squatting position, then the first two steps will be the same; to obtain the desired squat width, however, a third step should be taken out to the side with whichever foot the lifter feels most comfortable using. It may take a bit of practice to get into the proper stance in two or three steps, but, if practiced on every set from the first warm-up to the last heavy set, the lifter should master this skill in relatively little time. Unless you're a competitive power-lifter who competes in a federation that uses a monolift-style squat rack and you have one available to train with daily, you're going to need to walk the bar out from the racks before descending into your squat.

BREATHING

When executed properly, only one or two breaths need to be taken to execute a perfect squat, and this includes unracking the bar and set-ting up. Most lifters will find it preferable to take one breath before unracking the bar and setting up and another before descending into the squat. However, lifters who set up very efficiently and those us-ing a monolift are able to accomplish these two actions while taking a single breath. Lifters, after obtaining their grip and proper bar position but before unracking the bar, should take a deep breath, drawing the air deep into their stomach and pushing the abdominal muscles out against their belt to create tightness and stability. This is known as hoop tension and creates much more stability than breathing air into the chest and sucking the stomach inward, which is something that should be avoided. The breath is then held throughout the squat movement and only released after the lifter has pushed through the sticking point and is standing fully erect at the completion of the rep. Releasing the breath sooner will result in a loss of stability and increases the risk of injury. If performing sets of multiple reps, a breath would be released at the top of each rep, and a new one taken in and held before sitting back into the next squat descent.

BODYBUILDING VERSUS POWERLIFTING SQUATS

Powerlifters are only concerned with how much weight they can lift, and the more, the better. Thus the squat technique a powerlifter uses is designed to squat the most weight possible. It involves the most muscle groups possible and the best leverages to increase the amount of weight the athlete can squat. For these reasons and several others, many strength coaches feel this style of squatting is the most beneficial for athletes looking to increase their athletic performance. A powerlifting-style squat uses the hamstrings, glutes, erector muscles of the lower back, and the many small muscles of the hips to a greater degree than a bodybuilding-style squat, which tends to place the emphasis on the quadriceps muscles of the thighs. A powerlifting-style squat also places less stress on the knee joint because the shin is kept more vertical throughout the lift and the knee does not travel forward over the toes.

POWERLIFTING SQUAT TECHNIQUE

In a powerlifting-style squat, the first movement is back and not down, as most people would assume. First, the lifter's hips should move to the rear. To envision this properly, think of the motion used to sit back in a chair. While sitting back, the lifter should focus on keeping the chest up and the head facing straight forward. Failure to do so will cause the upper back to round, resulting in the lifter falling forward or in an excessive amount of stress being placed on the lower back muscles in order to complete the lift. As the lifter descends back and downward, the knees should be forced out. Many-times world champion, world record holder, and perhaps the greatest powerlifter of all time, Ed Coan, describes this as "opening your groin." As the lifter continues to sit back and nears parallel, the shins should be in a near vertical position. This technique not only provides the optimal leverage and helps engage all the necessary muscles but also greatly reduces the shearing forces on the patella tendons of the knee joint. Once the lifter has broken parallel, they should then explode upward, following the exact same groove that they descended in.

BODYBUILDING SQUAT TECHNIQUE

Since a bodybuilder's main goal in performing the squat is to add size to the quadriceps muscles of the upper thighs, a very different technique is required. The stance width will typically be much closer than a powerlifter's; shoulder width or slightly closer is the most common. While the same rules apply to grip, bar placement, setup, and breathing, the actual squatting motion is quite different than a powerlifter-style squat. Instead of sitting back, the lifter should sit down, and the knees should travel forward slightly and be kept pointing straight forward. Regardless of the technique used, the knees should never buckle inward, and the front of the knees should never go so far forward as to exceed the front of the toes, since this places a tremendous amount of stress onto the knee joint. The depth of the squat that is necessary when maximum quad development is the goal is debatable, and persuasive arguments can be made for squatting above parallel, to parallel, and even well below parallel. This should be determined by the individual lifter after experimenting with all three options, and some lifters may even find it beneficial to rotate between all three squat depths in their training.

PROGRAMMING THE SQUAT

Effective programming for the squat involves a well-planned progression in the amount of weight used, sufficiently addresses and prevents overtraining, stimulates hypertrophy, and reinforces proper technique. This program will not only significantly increase the amount the individual can squat but will also build new muscle mass.

The key to using this program effectively is starting with an accurate max. All too often, lifters overestimate their max or use a number they were previously capable of. It is essential to use your current true max that is obtained using proper form. Failure to do so will only result in overtraining and difficulty in progressing from week to week, negating the effectiveness of the program. In plain English: check your ego to make the most of this program. It is also important to note that the lifter's max is not to be recalculated at any point during the program. Strength increases have been factored into the design of this program, and adjusting the weights used during the program will decrease its effectiveness. This program is also designed for the athlete to squat only once every seven days. Attempting to train the squat more often than this following this program will quickly lead to an overtrained state and a reduction in strength.

16-WEEK WEIGHT PROGRESSION

WEEK 1	5 x 10 x 60% (5 sets of 10 reps at 60% of 1 rep max)
WEEK 2	5 x 8 x 65%
WEEK 3	5 x 5 x 70%
WEEK 4	5 x 3 x 75%
WEEK 5	5 x 10 x 60%
WEEK 6	5 x 8 x 70%
WEEK 7	5 x 5 x 75%
WEEK 8	5 x 3 x 80%
WEEK 9	5 x 10 x 60%
WEEK 10	4 x 8 x 75%
WEEK 11	4 x 5 x 80%
WEEK 12	4 x 3 x 85%
WEEK 13	5 x 10 x 60%
WEEK 14	3 x 8 x 80%
WEEK 15	3 x 5 x 85%
WEEK 16	3 x 3 x 90%

FIVE

USE BANDS TO BUILD SIZE AND STRENGTH

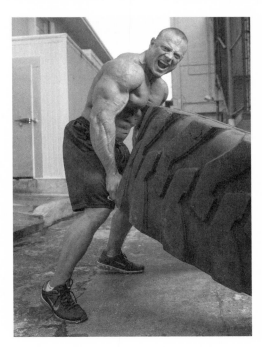

A BRIEF HISTORY AND INTRODUCTION

Two decades ago, no lifters had even heard of bands, let alone considered using them to augment their training. Thanks to Louie Simmons of Westside Barbell fame, they are now widely used. When properly implemented, their effectiveness has been well documented. Not only was Louie the first person to apply the bands to strength training, he also did a great deal to popularize their use. Through much analysis and experimentation, Louie designed many effective methods for their application. As a result, their popularity has spread into many other forms of athletics, and bands have been used not only to increase strength but also to aid in rehabbing injuries, to increase flexibility, and to develop explosiveness as it relates to athletics. However, many lifters still do not know how to properly implement bands into their training programs. I first incorporated bands into my training back in the late '90s and saw immediate results. Since then, I have experimented with a myriad of variations in their application for both powerlifting and bodybuilding purposes.

While bands can be used on their own as a source of resistance, I have found them to be most effective when combined with traditional barbell weight for basic compound movements. The bands come in a large variety of strengths and sizes, ranging from what is typically called a micro-mini band with a diameter of approximately 0.25 inches up to the strong bands that are up to 3.25 inches wide. Obviously, the amount of resistance provided is in direct proportion to the size of the band, and different sizes are appropriate for different uses. While I could probably write another book devoted to the best applications for the different sizes of bands, here I want to focus on one method of using the bands to increase the squat, bench, and deadlift while adding lots of lean muscle mass. This method is commonly referred to as the lightened method, or using reverse bands. Many of the top powerlifters in the world frequently use bands in this manner in their training.

APPLYING BANDS TO YOUR TRAINING

For powerlifters, or anyone looking to increase their strength, using the reverse band method provides several benefits. It allows the lifter to handle more weight than would otherwise be possible, which provides physiological and psychological benefits. Just being able to put more weight on your back or in your hands conditions you mentally to be able to lift those same weights in the future without the aid of the bands. The bands also adjust the force curve to work more efficiently with your body's natural leverages. What I mean by this is that the load you are lifting is decreased in the portion of the lift where your leverages are poorest (typically in the bottom part of the movement) and increased where your leverages are best (near lockout). This not only mimics the force curve for a competitive powerlifter who uses supportive gear like bench shirts and squat suits but also serves to substantially strengthen the musculature needed in the lockout portion of the lift. Even noncompetitive lifters often struggle most with the lockout of their bench presses and deadlifts, and it can be strongly argued that there is no better method for fixing that problem than incorporating the use of the reverse band method.

For bodybuilders, or anyone looking to add more lean muscle, the reverse band method provides additional benefits. It allows the lifter to handle greater loads while placing less stress on the muscles, joints, and connective tissue when they are in the most vulnerable positions of the movement. Most pec tears from bench-pressing happen when the bar is at the lifter's chest. For this reason, many pros do not lower the bar all the way to their chest or avoid bench-pressing altogether. With reverse-band bench-pressing, the load is lightened most while the bar is at the chest, minimizing the risk of a pec tear or shoulder injury. For squatting, again the load is lightened most in the bottom portion of the lift, when the stress on the hip joints and knees is greatest. I have used the reverse band method with great success when returning from both hip and knee injuries, when traditional squatting was not an option. The other major benefit of the reverse band method for bodybuilders is that, since the greatest loads occur near lockout and are minimized in the bottom portion of the lift, the emphasis is placed on the quadriceps and removed from the glutes and musculature of the hips. For lifters who need added leg size and do not wish to increase their glute size or strength, reverse band squatting can be an extremely beneficial movement.

HOW TO SET UP THE BANDS PROPERLY

When performing the squat, bench, or deadlift and using the reverse band method, it is easiest to do so inside a traditional power rack. Using a pair of bands of the same strength, attach one to each side of the power rack. by looping the bands around the top bars of the power rack and back through themselves in a slipknot. The open end is then pulled down and looped around each end of the barbell outside the plates. Collars will not be needed when setting up the bands with this method since the bands will act as collars themselves. Depending on the height of the power rack, the bands can also be looped around the safety bars, which should be placed in the higher holes of the rack if the rack is too high. And, of course, the bands can also be attached to any other secure overhead structure, as long as the height is sufficient and you are 100 percent confident that the structure can support the weight the bands will be applying. Powerlifters frequently attach the bands to the top of the monolift when squatting, which also works very well.

For bench-pressing and squatting, the bands can usually be set at the same or near the same height, but for deadlifting . the bands should be set up so that the bar would leave the bands if the bar were to travel past the lifter's belly button. The common mistake many lifters make when setting the bands up for the deadlift is either placing the bands too high (i.e., from the top of the power rack), thus providing far too much aid to the lift, or setting the bands up too low, where the bar actually leaves the bands before lockout. Many powerlifters employ the latter method, believing that having no aid from the bands at the top of the movement will actually further strengthen their lockout. However, what I have found is that this setup tends to alter lifters' technique and that their form often breaks down when trying to finish the lift, which, at worst, can lead to injury and, at best, will hinder their strength development.

One word of caution: when setting up your bands, be certain that the bands are not being pinched between the plates, bars, or equipment and that they are not being stretched or pulled across any sharp edges or rough surfaces. This will lead to the fraying of the bands and possible breakage, which could, of course, potentially subject the lifter to a severe injury.

WHAT BANDS TO USE FOR DIFFERENT-LEVEL LIFTERS

Below, I provide general guidelines for what strength of bands to use for different levels, but keep in mind that these are generalizations and that there may be exceptions based on the different variables of each lifter, such as overall height, limb length, and individual leverages. There are also many different techniques and methods of using the bands, and what I am describing here is just one variation. The bands I refer to are forty-one inches long, are typically made from latex, are one continuous loop without seams, and are flat, not hollow. Think of a giant rubber band, not the hollow rubber tubing sometimes passed off as bands made for lifting. Generally speaking, for reverse band benching, if your maximum bench press (without a bench shirt) is less than 300 pounds, you will find it most beneficial to use the light bands (1.125 inches wide). For a lifter capable of bench-pressing from 300 to 500 pounds, the medium bands (1.75 inches) are usually the best choice. For elite-level lifters who bench over 500 pounds raw, the strong bands (2.5 inches) typically provide the most optimal force curve. For squatting, I would recommend the light bands for anyone with a max squat of less than 405, the medium bands for those who squat between 405 and 600, and the strong bands for the elite-level lifters who are capable of squatting over 600 raw. For deadlifting, I generally recommend the light bands for anyone deadlifting less than 405, the medium bands for any lifter who pulls between 405 and 700, and the strong bands for lifters capable of dead-lifting over 700 pounds. The bands are available for purchase through www.elitefts.com and can be bought in pairs or as complete sets.

THE PROGRAM

What follows is a sixteen-week program that effectively uses the re-verse band method. While the strength of the bands and the resistance applied remain constant from week to week, the bar weight will be manipulated through four minicycles to induce both size and strength gains. This is designed not as a pure powerlifting- or bodybuilding-style program but rather for a lifter who desires to increase their muscle size and strength at the same time. This program is also not designed for someone who trains in powerlifting gear, and it should be performed without the aid of such equipment. You will notice that every fourth week is a week of five sets of ten reps, or what is some-times referred to as a "light" or "down" week. The purpose of this week is to allow recovery between the cycles of heavier weights and to pump the muscles full of blood with the high rep range, but don't mistakenly think this will be an easy week, because, as you will quickly see, it will not be easy at all.

THE MATH

The percentages are based on the maximum amount you can lift for a single repetition performed in the reverse band style. Before beginning the program, either find your true max by warming up thoroughly and then working up to a max reverse-band single (the use of spotters is highly recommended here) or work up to a single-set, 10-repetition maximum and use that number as 80 percent of your max, basing your other calculations on that. For example, let's say your 10-rep max on the reverse band bench is 320 pounds. Since $320 \div .8 = 400$, the max you would base your numbers on is 400. You would then perform week one at $5 \times 10 \times 240$ ($400 \times .6$), week two at $5 \times 8 \times 280$ ($400 \times .7$), week three at $5 \times 5 \times 300$ ($400 \times .75$), week four at $5 \times 3 \times 320$ ($400 \times .8$), and so on, according to the prescribed percentages.

16-WEEK WEIGHT PROGRESSION

WEEK 1	5 x 10 x 60% (5 sets of 10 reps at 60% of 1 rep max)
WEEK 2	5 x 8 x 70%
WEEK 3	5 x 5 x 75%
WEEK 4	5 x 3 x 80%
WEEK 5	5 x 10 x 60%
WEEK 6	5 x 8 x 75%
WEEK 7	5 x 5 x 80%
WEEK 8	5 x 3 x 85%
WEEK 9	5 x 10 x 60%
WEEK 10	4 x 8 x 80%
WEEK 11	4 x 5 x 85%
WEEK 12	4 x 3 x 90%
WEEK 13	5 x 10 x 60%
WEEK 14	3 x 8 x 85%
WEEK 15	3 x 5 x 90%
WEEK 16	3 x 3 x 95%

ALTERNATIVE STRENGTH-GAIN PROGRAM USING BANDS

For those primarily interested in increasing their strength, there is another program for using the reverse band method that I've had a lot of success with as well. The training cycle for this program is also designed in three-week waves, and every fourth week is a deload week. However, this time the strength of the bands is changed every four weeks. The program starts with the strongest bands and decreases the strength of the bands progressively every four weeks until, in the final cycle, the lifter is back to using only bar weight. This can be an extremely taxing training cycle because of the amount of weight used, so following the deload weeks exactly as described here is essential to avoiding overtraining and to reaping the maximum benefit from the program.

STRENGTH-TRAINING CYCLE FOR BENCH, SQUATS, AND DEADS USING BANDS

WEEK 1	(strong band) reverse band, work up to 5-rep max in 3-5 work sets
WEEK 2	(strong band) reverse band, work up to 3-rep max in 3-5 work sets
WEEK 3	(strong band) reverse band, work up to 1-rep max in 3-5 work sets
WEEK 4	(deload) bench and squats at 3 x 10 at 50% of raw max, no deadlifts
WEEK 5	(medium band) reverse band, work up to 5-rep max in 3-5 work sets
WEEK 6	(medium band) reverse band, work up to 3-rep max in 3-5 work sets
WEEK 7	(medium band) reverse band, work up to 1-rep max in 3-5 work sets
WEEK 8	(deload) bench and squats 3 x 10 at 50% of raw max, no deadlifts
WEEK 9	(light band) reverse band, work up to 5-rep max in 3-5 work sets
WEEK 10	(light band) reverse band, work up to 3-rep max in 3-5 work sets
WEEK 11	(light band) reverse band, work up to 1-rep max in 3-5 work sets

WEEK 12	(deload) bench and squats 3 x 10 at 50% of raw max, no deadlifts
WEEK 13	(no bands) work up to 5-rep max, in 3-5 work sets
WEEK 14	(no bands) work up to 3-rep max, in 3-5 work sets
WEEK 15	(no bands) work up to 1 rep max, in 3-5 work sets

SIX
KROC ROWS

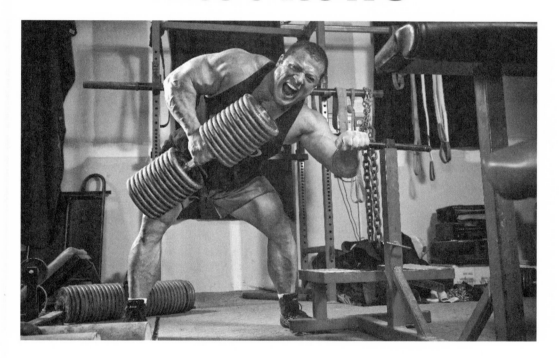

HISTORY

I don't think any book I'm writing can be complete without including a section about the exercise that I was fortunate enough to have named after me. Back in college, I began performing heavy dumbbell rows but never realized how important they were in my training until I stopped doing them. In 2002 I graduated from college, bought a new home, and moved several hours away to start a new job and raise my family. Because of the move, I had to start training in a commercial gym for the first time in years. Inadvertently, I stopped doing the heavy dumbbell rows in favor of using some of the new equipment I now had available to me. About a month before the 2002 USAPL Nationals, I went to pull some heavy deads to evaluate where my strength was at. For the first time in my competitive career, I had the bar slip from my hands on every one of my heavy singles. I was pulling around seven hundred pounds at the time and had never had grip issues in my life, so it befuddled me when I couldn't hang on to the bar at lockout for a heavy single. I was ripping the bar from the floor, only to have it peel its way out of my hands near the top. After that training session, I went home and tried to figure out what had changed in my training that would account for such a dramatic loss of grip strength. I pored over my training logs for the previous several months and realized that the only thing I had really changed was to stop doing dumbbell rows. I quickly added them back in, and at nationals a month later I went nine for nine and pulled all three deads with no grip issues.

From that point on, I was committed to keeping heavy dumbbell rows as a part of my training. The gym I was training at only had dumbbells up to 150 pounds, so I began going for rep records since I couldn't increase the weight. This was what first led to my performing sets of twenty to thirty reps without straps in this style. Later, I began putting together my own garage gym, so I went looking for the biggest dumbbells I could find. I was able to find a pair of handles that I could squeeze 225 pounds onto by using vise grips as collars. Around this time, I was knocking the 225s out for sets of twenty-five reps, and my upper-back strength and size were increasing significantly. Another thing I noticed was that the previous problem I had with locking out my deadlifts had disappeared, and now I was able to easily finish any pull that I could get to my knees. It was around this time that I became part of the Elitefts.com team and traveled to London, Ohio, to train at the compound with Dave Tate and Jim Wendler for the first time. During that training session, I performed a set of dumbbell rows for 225 × 25, and afterward Wendler asked me why I was doing them and how I believed they helped me. I explained to him that they had vastly improved my grip strength and had added significant size and strength to my upper back, which had improved my deadlift lockout. After giving them a try himself, Jim recommended the rows to some other powerlifters that he knew, and all of them noticed an immediate improvement in both their grip and upper back strength, which also carried over to their deadlift maxes. Jim began referring to this exercise as "Kroc rows," and that's how they came to be known. A little while later, after searching without success for larger dumbbell handles, I approached my brother, who is an ironworker, about making a custom pair of handles that could hold in excess of three hundred pounds. My brother ended up finding a pair of thirty-six-inch-long, double-threaded bolts that were actually made for anchoring large buildings. They were made from hardened steel and were long enough and strong enough to hold the amount of weight I needed. My brother welded some inside collars onto them, and I began working toward the three-hundred-pound rows that I am now known for. As a result of frequent questions from lifters looking for their own set of dumbbell handles with which to do Kroc rows, I partnered with a manufacturer to produce very high-quality Kroc Row Dumbbell Handles that hold well over three hundred pounds each and are virtually indestructible. They can be purchased at www.mattkroc.com. Not coincidentally, when I began really increasing the weight and reps on this exercise, my deadlift climbed from the low to mid seven hundreds to over eight hundred pounds, all while remaining in the 220-pound class.

BENEFITS

As mentioned previously, Kroc rows can add slabs of muscle to your upper back and forearms and dramatically increase your grip and upper-back strength, helping anyone attempting to increase their deadlift. Performing them without using straps for high-rep ranges will work your forearms and grip strength better than anything else I have tried. The high-rep ranges combined with heavy weights are also great for adding lots of thickness and width to your upper back. My back is my strongest body part on the bodybuilding stage, and Kroc rows are the primary reason why. Doing them with really heavy weights will also strengthen your upper back like nothing else, allowing you to lockout any weight you can pull to your knees. Of course, this exercise doesn't just offer significant benefit to bodybuilders and powerlifters but to strongman competitors or anyone looking for strength that carries over well to lifting and moving heavy objects in everyday life. I've used my back strength to carry engine blocks, furniture, washers, and even a fully loaded refrigerator all by myself. There is no doubt that possessing a very strong upper back will make you much more powerful not only in the gym but also in the real world.

PROPER TECHNIQUE

Anyone who has ever watched me perform a Kroc row or given one a try themselves knows right away that this is not the dumbbell row that your spandex-wearing, buck-o-five weighing, certified personal trainer has taught you how to do. There is no pulling back in an arc or squeezing at the top while holding a shiny chrome fifteen-pound dumbbell. No, Kroc rows are all about heavy weight, high reps, plenty of sweat, and sometimes even a little blood.

While the form may be somewhat looser than your standard row, don't believe for a minute that you won't be working the desired muscles. Simply put: anyone would be hard-pressed to move a weight from arm's length to their chest in a bent-over position without using the upper back musculature to a significant degree. Those are simply the muscles that must be used to move a weight in that fashion. However, I don't want you to think that form doesn't matter, because there are a couple key technique points that must be followed to get the greatest benefit possible from Kroc rows.

The first thing you need to concentrate on is getting a full range of motion by fully extending the shoulder at the bottom of the movement and really pulling it up and back at the top of the movement. This will ensure a full stretch in the lats in the bottom position and a complete contraction at the top. At the bottom, really let your shoulder drop; you should feel the stretch in your lats and middle-upper back. At the top, concentrate on retracting your scapula as far back as possible as you pull your elbow up and back, essentially trying to squeeze your shoulder blades together. Your shoulders should be kept higher than your hips and your upper back should be at approximately a fifteen-degree angle in relation to the floor. Think of putting an adjustable incline bench on the lowest setting: that is the angle you are shooting for. This angle will focus the movement primarily on your upper back. The dumbbell should be pulled in a straight line from directly below your chest up to the lower portion of your rib cage. I make it a point to lightly touch the dumbbell to my rib cage at the top of every rep. A little bit of body English is acceptable, but don't use momentum to make the movement easier. Explode the weight up using your upper back muscles, but do not do it in a clean-type motion that will use momentum to move the weight, since this will reduce the amount of work your muscles are required to do.

You can perform Kroc rows with one hand and one knee on a flat bench or standing with your nonrowing hand braced on something solid that will allow you to maintain the proper angle of your upper back. You can post your hand on the end of a dumbbell rack, a different piece of equipment, or any solid structure that allows you to stabilize your body but still provides clearance for the large dumbbell. Once I started using dumbbells that weighed in excess of 225 pounds, the three-foot-long dumbbells were too long to use on a regular bench without making contact with it, so I had to perform the rows using the standing technique.

Contrary to popular belief, Kroc rows can be performed with wrist straps. In fact, I often rotate back and forth between performing them with and without straps. Obviously, performing them without straps is an excellent way to increase your grip strength. But if your focus is on building upper back strength and size, it is perfectly acceptable to use straps from time to time to allow you to handle the most weight possible. While I have done 40 reps with 175 pounds and 30 reps with 205 pounds without straps, there is no way I could have hit my PR (personal record) of 13 reps with 300 pounds without throwing the straps on. Using the straps allows me to focus on my upper back and to hit it with the most weight and intensity possible without having to worry about my grip failing. I believe it is best to rotate between both styles to reap the greatest rewards possible from Kroc rows. I often simply perform them one week with straps and then the next week without and rotate back and forth on a weekly basis.

Regarding set and rep structure, I have found the benefits of Kroc rows to be greatest when working up to one set to failure. I typically perform two to three warm-up sets and then go all out for one max set, attempting to hit either a weight or rep PR every time I perform them. I recommend shooting for at least twenty reps and not increasing the weight until you can get at least twenty-five reps with each arm. I have gone as high as forty reps per set, and my back was pumped beyond belief afterward. Performing Kroc rows with heavy weights and high reps will leave you gasping for air like a drop set of heavy squats. They are definitely not for the weak minded or faint hearted. If you really want to get the most out of Kroc rows, you need to dig down deep and keep going until you truly reach complete muscular exhaustion, which most lifters think they reach at the end of a set, but few actually do.

SUMMARY

1. Ensure a full range of motion by fully extending the shoulder at the bottom of the movement and really pulling it up and back at the top.
2. Your shoulders should be kept higher than your hips and your upper back should be at approximately a fifteen-degree angle in relation to the floor.
3. Row the dumbbell in a straight line from directly below your chest up to the lower portion of your rib cage.
4. You can perform Kroc rows with one hand and one knee on a flat bench or standing with your nonrowing hand braced on something solid.
5. Rotate back and forth between performing Kroc rows with and without straps to reap the most benefit from the movement.
6. After two to three warm-up sets, go all out for one max set, attempting to hit either a weight or rep PR every time you perform them, shooting for at least twenty reps per set.
7. Perform Kroc rows with as much weight as possible and strive to go to complete muscular failure on the final set.

Follow these key technique points, use as much weight as physically possible, go until you reach complete muscular exhaustion, and watch both your back strength and size increase like never before.

SEVEN
THE THOUSAND-REP ARM-TRAINING SESSION

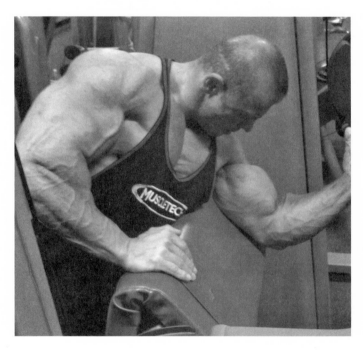

Probably the most challenging arm-training session I've ever done was designed to increase arm size in individuals for whom nothing else has worked or who have been stuck at a certain size for a long time. The technique is not meant to be used every week but rather about once a month—to shock the muscles into growth with extreme volume. Performing it any more frequently than that is likely to lead to overtraining and regression, because the overall volume of work is so incredibly high for these relatively small muscle groups. It is comprised of ten exercises, all of which are five sets of twenty reps. It is okay to lighten the weights somewhat after the first few exercises to ensure you get all of the reps. The priority here is completing every set and every rep inside the prescribed rest periods and not the amount of weight used.

EZ-BAR CURLS: After a few warm-up sets, perform five sets of twenty reps with two to three minutes of rest between sets.

STRAIGHT BAR PUSHDOWNS: After a few warm-up sets, perform 5 sets of 20 reps with 2–3 minutes of rest between sets. Keep your elbows glued to your sides and don't pause the reps; just pump them up and down.

CABLE CURLS: Use an EZ-curl-shaped handle and attach it to the lower cable. Perform 5 sets of 20 reps with 2–3 minutes of rest between sets.

OVERHEAD CABLE EXTENSIONS: Use a rope handle attached to the high pulley. Face away from the machine and bend over at the waist, extending the rope from behind your head straight out in front of you to arm's length. Perform 5 sets of 20 reps with 2–3 minutes of rest between sets.

DUMBBELL HAMMER CURLS: Keep your elbows at your sides and perform all the reps with both arms at the same time. Perform 5 sets of 20 reps with 2–3 minutes of rest between sets.

LYING EXTENSIONS WITH CHAINS: Lie flat on your back and perform a skull-crusher-type movement with chains. These can be with an EZ-curl bar, with the chains clipped to D handles or the grenade handles from Elitefts.com if you have them. Perform 5 sets of 20 reps with 2–3 minutes of rest between sets.

SEATED BARBELL CURLS: Use a straight barbell for these and perform them strictly, touching your thighs at the bottom of the movement but not resting the weight on them. Perform 5 sets of 20 reps with 2–3 minutes of rest between sets.

DUMBBELL KICKBACKS: Bend over at the waist and extend both arms at the same time. Keep your upper arms parallel to the floor and pause the reps briefly at the top with full extension while flexing the triceps. Perform 5 sets of 20 reps with only 1–2 minutes of rest between sets.

EZ-BAR REVERSE CURLS: Keep your form strict here and limit the amount of body swing, using lighter weights if necessary since your arms should be completely fried by this point. Perform 5 sets of 20 reps with 2–3 minutes of rest between sets.

BENCH DIPS: Body weight is all you should need by the time you get here. Set up two benches of the same height. Perform dips in between them, keeping your legs straight, your feet on one bench, and your hands on the bench just behind you. Perform 5 sets of 20 reps with only 1–2 minutes of rest between sets.

EIGHT

REVERSE-PYRAMID FOR STRENGTH AND SIZE

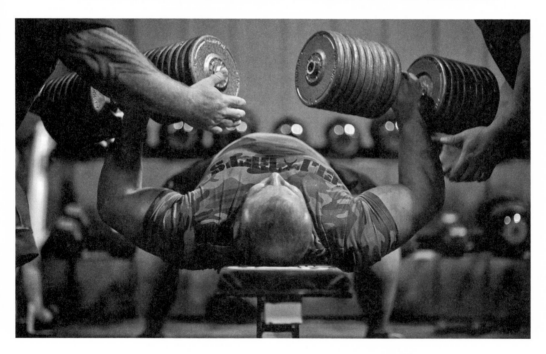

The methodology for this program is based on linear periodization but with a key alteration. Instead of just a steady progression in the amount of weight used, there is a wave system built into the program. The reason for this waving, or undulation, in intensity is twofold. It prevents overtraining by providing periodic deloads at key intervals, and it also allows for greater length of time of progression in the amount of weight lifted. If you were to just steadily increase the amount of weight used from week to week, it wouldn't be long before your progress stalled. The wave technique provides us with the ability to continually progress for a much longer period of time before we reach a plateau.

There is an additional unusual element to this program. The main exercises (squats, benches, and deadlifts) are performed by inverting the relationship between set and intensity progression. Stated plainly: as the sets progress, there is a small decrease in the amount of weight used, instead of the usual increase. The purpose of this is to allow the lifter to perform every set in good form and to ensure that the lifter never misses a rep in training, even as the amount of weight increases from week to week. Contrary to popular belief, training to failure and beyond is not always desirable when trying to build strength. When programmed properly, not missing reps in training can be a key ingredient to building strength—and as we know, gaining strength is a vital component to gaining size.

The exercise selection is based largely on multijoint compound movements. As many of you probably already know, these types of exercises allow us to use more weight, which in turn yields greater muscle-fiber recruitment, which ultimately leads to a greater degree of muscular hypertrophy. Another key element to gaining mass is ensuring a large volume of blood is being forced into the muscle while training. More commonly known as the "pump" because of the way your muscles swell while lifting, the pump is often synonymous with an increase in muscle size. A good pump stretches the connective tissue that surrounds the muscle fibers, allowing room for new growth. Arnold was often quoted as saying that a good pump means you're growing, and he was right. This program achieves a massive pump both through overall training volume (a relatively high number of sets and/or reps) and through specific exercises done for higher rep ranges with shorter rest periods. For example, dumbbell rows, front squats, and barbell shrugs are all performed for sets of twenty reps but are still performed with relatively heavy weights, which, when combined with minimal rest periods, provides us with a high volume of blood being forced into the muscle. There are other methods used to achieve this, like the shoulder complex, which is a triset of three different exercises, all performed back-to-back without rest. By the end of your third triset, your shoulders will be blown up like balloons.

You will be training five days a week, and Thursday and Sunday will be the off days. Splitting things up into five days allows us to hit the individual muscles with sufficient volume during the training session without doing marathon workouts. The order of the individual training sessions ensures that there will be sufficient recovery time before the same muscles are trained again. It breaks down like this:

MONDAY: LOWER BACK, HAMSTRINGS, AND CALVES
TUESDAY: CHEST AND SHOULDERS
WEDNESDAY: UPPER BACK
THURSDAY: OFF
FRIDAY: LEGS
SATURDAY: BICEPS AND TRICEPS
SUNDAY: OFF

After warming up, deadlifts, bench presses, and squats are performed for five sets of five reps with the weight selection in accordance with the weight progression percentages listed at the end of this chapter. You will be required to find your maxes on these exercises before beginning this program so you can plug the correct numbers into the formula. One word of caution here: do not guess your maxes. Overestimating them will lead to an inability to achieve the desired number of reps and to overtraining, ultimately resulting in a failure of the entire program.

The wave technique comes into play with the main exercises (squats, bench presses, and deadlifts). The amount of weight used will increase over each three-week wave. The fourth week will consist of a deload week, during which the amount of weight used will be substantially decreased to facilitate recovery and prevent overtraining. Then, the next wave begins. However, don't be fooled into thinking that the deload weeks will be easy. While the amount of weight used decreases, the amount of reps performed doubles, ensuring that you will still be working hard and stimulating growth even while preventing overtraining. The overall program length is written for sixteen weeks, which is comprised of four waves. At the end of the sixteen weeks, you will then find your new maxes, and, if you desire, you can plug them back into the table and begin the program again.

Rest periods should be kept to no more than five minutes maximum on the large compound movements like squats, bench presses, and deadlifts and at no more than two to three minutes for more isolation-type exercises like spider curls and pushdowns. This will ensure adequate recovery between sets but still provide you with the huge pump that you are looking for. If you are able to achieve all of the desired reps in good form for the assistance movements (everything besides squats, bench presses, and deadlifts), increase the weight by a small amount for the following week. On these exercises, we are not as concerned about missing an occasional rep because of achieving muscular failure as we are for squats, bench presses, and deadlifts.

TRAINING PROGRAM

MONDAY: LOWER BACK, HAMS, AND CALVES

DEADLIFTS: warm up, then follow weight progression at the end of the chapter

PULL THROUGHS: 3×20

LYING LEG CURLS: 2×10

SEATED OR STANDING LEG CURLS: 2×10

ANY TYPE OF CALF RAISE: 4×25

TUESDAY: CHEST AND SHOULDERS

BENCH PRESSES: warm up, then follow weight progression at the end of the chapter

INCLINE PRESSES: pyramid up in weight sets of 12, 10, 8, 6

DIPS: pyramid up in weight sets of 15, 12, 10, 8

STANDING MILITARY PRESS: pyramid up in weight sets of 10, 8, 6

SHOULDER COMPLEX: do 20 front raises, 20 lateral raises, and 20 bent laterals; use dumbbells and perform one continuous set, moving immediately from one exercise to the next; repeat 3 times

WEDNESDAY: UPPER BACK

HEAVY DUMBBELL ROWS: 2×20, go as heavy on these as possible

CHINS: 50 reps total with body weight, in as many sets as it takes; rotate between 2 to 3 different grips

T-BAR ROWS: pyramid up in weight sets of 12, 10, 8, 6

LAT PULL-DOWNS: pyramid up in weight sets of 15, 12, 10, 8

BARBELL SHRUGS: 2×20 reps, as heavy as possible

FRIDAY: LEGS

SQUATS: warm up, then follow weight progression at the end of the chapter

LEG PRESSES: pyramid up in weight for sets of 15, 12, 10, 8

FRONT SQUATS: 2×20

WALKING LUNGES: 2×30 steps

ANY TYPE OF CALF RAISE: 4×25

SATURDAY: BICEPS AND TRICEPS

CLOSE-GRIP BENCH: pyramid up in weight sets of 10, 8, 6

SKULL CRUSHERS: pyramid up in weight sets of 12, 10, 8

PUSHDOWNS: pyramid up in weight sets of 15, 12, 10

BENCH DIPS: 3×20

BARBELL CURLS: pyramid up in weight sets of 15, 12, 10

PREACHER CURLS: pyramid up in weight sets of 15, 12, 10
DUMBBELL INCLINE CURLS: pyramid up in weight sets of 15, 12, 10
DUMBBELL SPIDER CURLS: 3×20

WEIGHT PROGRESSION FOR SQUATS, BENCH PRESSES, AND DEADLIFTS

WEEK 1	5 x 80%, 5 x 77.5%, 5 x 75%, 5 x 72.5%, 5 x 70%
WEEK 2	5 x 82.5%, 5 x 80%, 5 x 77.5%, 5 x 75%, 5 x 72.5%
WEEK 3	5 x 85%, 5 x 82.5%, 5 x 80%, 5 x 77.5%, 5 x 75%
WEEK 4	deload, squats and bench presses 5 x 10 at 60%; no deadlifts
WEEK 5	5 x 82.5%, 5 x 80%, 5 x 77.5%, 5 x 75%, 5 x 72.5%
WEEK 6	5 x 85%, 5 x 82.5%, 5 x 80%, 5 x 77.5%, 5 x 75%
WEEK 7	5 x 87.5%, 5 x 85%, 5 x 82.5%, 5 x 80%, 5 x 77.5%
WEEK 8	deload, squats and bench presses 5 x 10 at 60%; no deadlifts
WEEK 9	5 x 85%, 5 x 82.5%, 5 x 80%, 5 x 77.5%, 5 x 75%
WEEK 10	5 x 87.5%, 5 x 85%, 5 x 82.5%, 5 x 80%, 5 x 77.5%
WEEK 11	5 x 90%, 5 x 87.5%, 5 x 85%, 5 x 82.5%, 5 x 80%
WEEK 12	deload, squats and bench presses 5 x 10 at 60%; no deadlifts
WEEK 13	5 x 87.5%, 5 x 85%, 5 x 82.5%, 5 x 80%, 5 x 77.5%
WEEK 14	5 x 90%, 5 x 87.5%, 5 x 85%, 5 x 82.5%, 5 x 80%
WEEK 15	5 x 92.5%, 5 x 90%, 5 x 87.5%, 5 x 85%, 5 x 82.5%
WEEK 16	deload, squats and bench presses 5 x 10 x 60%; no deadlifts
WEEK 17	find new maxes on squat, bench presses, and deads

NINE

OFF-SEASON POWERLIFTING FOR GEARED LIFTERS

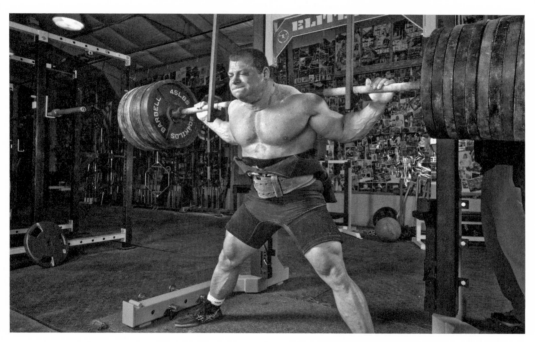

This program is designed for competitive powerlifters who compete wearing powerlifting gear. It is to be used when not prepping for a meet to promote off-season strength gains. On all heavy squats, benches, and deadlifts, work up to your goal for each day, but do NOT miss reps, only taking weights you know you can get. Work very hard and come as close as you can to your true max, but err on the side of caution and leave a rep in the tank if necessary but do NOT miss.

I emphasize this since it is imperative to the success of the program and will help prevent overtraining as well as promote strength gains.

FIRST CYCLE

WEEK ONE

FRIDAY

SQUATS: work up to max triple in full gear
FRONT SQUATS: 3 sets of 10 reps
PULL-THROUGHS: 3 sets of 20 reps
GLUTE/HAM RAISES OR HYPERS: 3 sets of 20 reps
CALF RAISES (ANY STYLE): 3 sets of 25 reps

SATURDAY

BENCH: reverse band presses with blue bands, work up to max triple
DUMBBELL BENCH: 3 sets of 10 reps
CHINS: do 50 reps total in as many sets as it takes
SEATED DUMBBELL POWER CLEANS: 3 sets of 20 reps
PUSHDOWNS: 3 sets of 10 reps

MONDAY

DEADLIFTS: partials with plates 6 inches off ground, work up to max single
DUMBBELL ROWS: 2 sets of 20 reps, as heavy as possible
T-BAR ROWS: work up to heavy set of 10 reps
BARBELL SHRUGS: work up to heavy set of 10 reps in 3–4 sets
BARBELL CURLS: 3 sets of 10 reps

TUESDAY

STANDING MILITARY PRESS: work up to heavy triple

CLOSE-GRIP BENCH: work up to heavy set of 10 in 3–4 sets

SEATED DUMBBELL POWER CLEANS: 3 sets of 20 reps

DIPS: do 50 reps total in as many sets as it takes

WEEK TWO

FRIDAY

SQUATS, REVERSE BLUE BAND: work up to max triple in briefs or suit bottoms only

FRONT SQUATS: 3 sets of 10 reps

PULL-THROUGHS: 3 sets of 20 reps

GLUTE/HAM RAISES OR HYPERS: 3 sets of 20 reps

CALF RAISES (ANY STYLE): 3 sets of 25 reps

SATURDAY

BENCH: 3-board presses—work up to max triple

DUMBBELL BENCH: 3 sets of 10 reps

CHINS: do 50 reps total in as many sets as it takes

SEATED DUMBBELL POWER CLEANS: 3 sets of 20 reps

PUSHDOWNS: 3 sets of 10 reps

MONDAY

DEADLIFTS: Partials with plates 3 inches off ground, work up to max single

DUMBBELL ROWS: 2 sets of 20 reps, as heavy as possible

T-BAR ROWS: work up to heavy set of 10 reps

BARBELL SHRUGS: work up to heavy set of 10 reps in 3–4 sets

BARBELL CURLS: 3 sets of 10 reps

TUESDAY

SEATED MILITARY PRESS: work up to heavy triple

CLOSE-GRIP BENCH: work up to heavy set of 10 in 3–4 sets

SEATED DUMBBELL POWER CLEANS: 3 sets of 20 reps

DIPS: do 50 reps total in as many sets as it takes

WEEK THREE

FRIDAY

SQUATS: work up to single in full gear

FRONT SQUATS: 3 sets of 10 reps

PULL-THROUGHS: 3 sets of 20 reps

GLUTE/HAM RAISES OR HYPERS: 3 sets of 20 reps

CALF RAISES (ANY STYLE): 3 sets of 25 reps

SATURDAY

BENCH, RAW: work up to max triple

DUMBBELL BENCH: 3 sets of 10 reps

CHINS: do 50 reps total in as many sets as it takes

SEATED DUMBBELL POWER CLEANS: 3 sets of 20 reps

PUSHDOWNS: 3 sets of 10 reps

MONDAY

DEADLIFTS: from the ground, work up to max single

DUMBBELL ROWS: 2 sets of 20 reps, as heavy as possible

T-BAR ROWS: work up to heavy set of 10 reps

BARBELL SHRUGS: work up to heavy set of 10 reps in 3–4 sets

BARBELL CURLS: 3 sets of 10 reps

TUESDAY

STANDING PUSH-PRESS: work up to heavy triple

CLOSE-GRIP BENCH: work up to heavy set of 10 in 3–4 sets

SEATED DUMBBELL POWER CLEANS: 3 sets of 20 reps

DIPS: do 50 reps total in as many sets as it takes

WEEK FOUR: DELOAD WEEK

FRIDAY

SQUATS OFF PARALLEL BOX: 8 sets of doubles at 50% of max using only straight weight, wearing belt and briefs (if no briefs, wear suit bottoms)

FRONT SQUATS: 3 sets of 10 reps

PULL-THROUGHS: 3 sets of 20 reps

GLUTE/HAM RAISES OR HYPERS: 3 sets of 20 reps

CALF RAISES (ANY STYLE): 3 sets of 25 reps

SATURDAY

BENCH: 3 sets of 15 reps at 60% of max

CHINS: do 50 reps total in as many sets as it takes

SEATED DUMBBELL POWER CLEANS: 3 sets of 20 reps

PUSHDOWNS: 3 sets of 10 reps

MONDAY (NO DEADLIFTS)

DUMBBELL ROWS: 2 sets of 20 reps, as heavy as possible

T-BAR ROWS: work up to heavy set of 10 reps

BARBELL SHRUGS: work up to heavy set of 10 reps in 3–4 sets

BARBELL CURLS: 3 sets of 10 reps

TUESDAY

SEATED DUMBBELL PRESSES: easy 3 sets of 10 reps

CLOSE-GRIP BENCH: 2 sets of 10 reps

SEATED DUMBBELL POWER CLEANS: 3 sets of 20 reps

DIPS: do 50 reps total in as many sets as it takes

SECOND CYCLE

WEEK ONE

FRIDAY

SQUATS, REVERSE GREEN BAND: work up to max triple in suit bottoms or briefs

FRONT SQUATS: 3 sets of 10 reps

PULL-THROUGHS: 3 sets of 20 reps

GLUTE/HAM RAISES OR HYPERS: 3 sets of 20 reps

CALF RAISES (ANY STYLE): 3 sets of 25 reps

SATURDAY

BENCH: five-board presses, work up to max triple

DUMBBELL BENCH: 3 sets of 10 reps

CHINS: do 50 reps total in as many sets as it takes

SEATED DUMBBELL POWER CLEANS: 3 sets of 20 reps

PUSHDOWNS: 3 sets of 10 reps

MONDAY

DEADLIFTS: work up to max set of 5 reps

DUMBBELL ROWS: 2 sets of 20 reps, as heavy as possible

T-BAR ROWS: work up to heavy set of 10 reps

BARBELL SHRUGS: work up to heavy set of 10 reps in 3–4 sets

BARBELL CURLS: 3 sets of 10 reps

TUESDAY

SEATED PRESSES: off pins in power rack, set height 1 inch above your head; work up to max triple

CLOSE-GRIP BENCH: work up to heavy set of 10 in 3–4 sets

SEATED DUMBBELL POWER CLEANS: 3 sets of 20 reps

DIPS: do 50 reps total in as many sets as it takes

MATT KROCZALESKI

WEEK TWO

FRIDAY

SQUATS, REVERSE BLUE BAND: work up to max triple in briefs or suit bottoms

FRONT SQUATS: 3 sets of 10 reps

PULL-THROUGHS: 3 sets of 20 reps

GLUTE/HAM RAISES OR HYPERS: 3 sets of 20 reps

CALF RAISES (ANY STYLE): 3 sets of 25 reps

SATURDAY

BENCH-FLOOR PRESSES: work up to max triple

DUMBBELL BENCH: 3 sets of 10 reps

CHINS: do 50 reps total in as many sets as it takes

SEATED DUMBBELL POWER CLEANS: 3 sets of 20 reps

PUSHDOWNS: 3 sets of 10 reps

MONDAY

DEADLIFTS: work up to max triple

DUMBBELL ROWS: 2 sets of 20 reps, as heavy as possible

T-BAR ROWS: work up to heavy set of 10 reps

BARBELL SHRUGS: work up to heavy set of 10 reps in 3–4 sets

BARBELL CURLS: 3 sets of 10 reps

TUESDAY

SEATED DUMBBELL PRESSES: work up to 5-rep max

CLOSE-GRIP BENCH: work up to heavy set of 10 in 3–4 sets

SEATED DUMBBELL POWER CLEANS: 3 sets of 20 reps

DIPS: do 50 reps total in as many sets as it takes

WEEK THREE

FRIDAY

SQUATS, REVERSE BLUE AND PINK BAND: work up to max triple in briefs or suit bottoms
FRONT SQUATS: 3 sets of 10 reps
PULL-THROUGHS: 3 sets of 20 reps
GLUTE/HAM RAISES OR HYPERS: 3 sets of 20 reps
CALF RAISES (ANY STYLE): 3 sets of 25 reps

SATURDAY

BENCH: reverse blue band presses, work up to max single
DUMBBELL BENCH: 3 sets of 10 reps
CHINS: do 50 reps total in as many sets as it takes
SEATED DUMBBELL POWER CLEANS: 3 sets of 20 reps
PUSHDOWNS: 3 sets of 10 reps

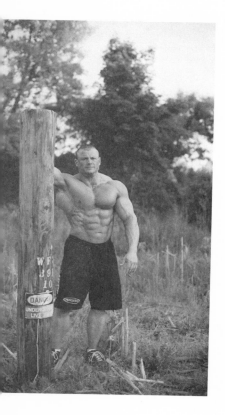

MONDAY

DEADLIFTS: work up to max single
DUMBBELL ROWS: 2 sets of 20 reps, as heavy as possible
T-BAR ROWS: work up to heavy set of 10 reps
BARBELL SHRUGS: work up to heavy set of 10 reps in 3–4 sets
BARBELL CURLS: 3 sets of 10 reps

TUESDAY

STANDING PUSH-PRESS: work up to heavy single
CLOSE-GRIP BENCH: work up to heavy set of 10 in 3–4 sets
SEATED DUMBBELL POWER CLEANS: 3 sets of 20 reps
DIPS: do 50 reps total in as many sets as it takes

WEEK FOUR: D WEEK

FRIDAY

SQUATS OFF PARALLEL BOX: 8 sets of doubles at 50% of max only using straight weight, wearing belt and briefs (if no briefs, wear suit bottoms)

FRONT SQUATS: 3 sets of 10 reps

PULL-THROUGHS: 3 sets of 20 reps

GLUTE/HAM RAISES OR HYPERS: 3 sets of 20 reps

CALF RAISES (ANY STYLE): 3 sets of 25 reps

SATURDAY

BENCH: 3 sets of 15 reps at 60% of max

CHINS: do 50 reps total in as many sets as it takes

SEATED DUMBBELL POWER CLEANS: 3 sets of 20 reps

PUSHDOWNS: 3 sets of 10 reps

MONDAY

(NO DEADLIFTS)

DUMBBELL ROWS: 2 sets of 20 reps, as heavy as possible

T-BAR ROWS: work up to heavy set of 10 reps

BARBELL SHRUGS: work up to heavy set of 10 reps in 3–4 sets

BARBELL CURLS: 3 sets of 10 reps

TUESDAY

SEATED DUMBBELL PRESSES: easy 3 sets of 10 reps

CLOSE-GRIP BENCH: 2 sets of 10 reps

SEATED DUMBBELL POWER CLEANS: 3 sets of 20 reps

DIPS: 50 reps total in as many sets as it takes

THIRD CYCLE

WEEK ONE

FRIDAY

BOX SQUATS: in briefs, 6 sets of doubles with pink (light) bands pulling down (use a weight you think you could do 10 times in briefs without the bands)

WALKING LUNGES: 3 sets of 20 steps

PULL-THROUGHS: 3 sets of 20 reps

GLUTE/HAM RAISES OR HYPERS: 3 sets of 20 reps

CALF RAISES (ANY STYLE): 3 sets of 25 reps

SATURDAY

REVERSE BAND PRESSES WITH BLUE BAND: work up to 5-rep max

WEIGHTED DIPS (LEAN FORWARD TO EMPHASIZE CHEST): 3 sets of 10 reps

LAT PULLS: work up to heavy set of 6 in a pyramid fashion over 3–4 sets

SEATED DUMBBELL POWER CLEANS: 3 sets of 20 reps

PUSHDOWNS (IF YOU HAVE BEEN USING A BAR, SWITCH TO ROPE OR VICE VERSA): 3 sets of 10 reps

MONDAY

REVERSE BLUE-BAND DEADLIFTS (HANG BAND FROM TOP OF POWER CAGE): work up to 5-rep max

DUMBBELL ROWS: 2 sets of 10 reps, as heavy as possible

T-BAR ROWS: work up to heavy set of 6 reps

BARBELL SHRUGS: work up to heavy set of 10 reps in 3–4 sets

DUMBBELL CURLS: 3 sets of 10 reps

TUESDAY

STANDING PUSH PRESS: work up to 5-rep max

CLOSE-GRIP BENCH: 3 work sets of 10, 8, and 6 reps, increasing weight each set

BARBELL, UPRIGHT ROWS: 3 work sets of 12, 10 and 8 reps increasing weight each set

BENCH DIPS (PLACE PLATES IN LAP): 3 sets of 10 reps

WEEK TWO

FRIDAY

BOX SQUATS, IN BRIEFS: 6 sets of doubles with green (medium) bands pulling down (use same bar weight as previous week)

WALKING LUNGES: 3 sets of 20 steps

PULL-THROUGHS: 3 sets of 20 reps

GLUTE/HAM RAISES OR HYPERS: 3 sets of 20 reps

CALF RAISES (ANY STYLE): 3 sets of 25 reps

SATURDAY

REVERSE BAND PRESSES WITH BLUE BAND: work up to 3-rep max

WEIGHTED DIPS (LEAN FORWARD TO EMPHASIZE CHEST): 3 sets of 10 reps

LAT PULLS: work up to heavy set of 6 in a pyramid fashion over 3–4 sets

SEATED DUMBBELL POWER CLEANS: 3 sets of 20 reps

PUSHDOWNS (IF YOU HAVE BEEN USING A BAR, SWITCH TO ROPE OR VICE VERSA): 3 sets of 10 reps

MONDAY

REVERSE BLUE-BAND DEADLIFTS (HANG BAND FROM TOP OF POWER CAGE): work up to 3-rep max

DUMBBELL ROWS: 2 sets of 10 reps, as heavy as possible

T-BAR ROWS: work up to heavy set of 6 reps

BARBELL SHRUGS: work up to heavy set of 10 reps in 3–4 sets

DUMBBELL CURLS: 3 sets of 10 reps

TUESDAY

STANDING PUSH PRESS: work up to 3-rep max

CLOSE-GRIP BENCH: 3 work sets of 10, 8, and 6 reps, increasing weight each set

BARBELL, UPRIGHT ROWS: 3 work sets of 12, 10, and 8 reps, increasing weight each set

BENCH DIPS (PLACE PLATES IN LAP): 3 sets of 10 reps

WEEK THREE

FRIDAY

BOX SQUATS, IN BRIEFS: 6 sets of doubles with blue bands, pulling down (use same bar weight as previous week)

WALKING LUNGES: 3 sets of 20 steps

PULL-THROUGHS: 3 sets of 20 reps

GLUTE/HAM RAISES OR HYPERS: 3 sets of 20 reps

CALF RAISES (ANY STYLE): 3 sets of 25 reps

SATURDAY

REVERSE BAND PRESSES WITH BLUE BAND: work up to max single

WEIGHTED DIPS (LEAN FORWARD TO EMPHASIZE CHEST): 3 sets of 10 reps

LAT PULLS: work up to heavy set of 6 in a pyramid fashion over 3–4 sets

SEATED DUMBBELL POWER CLEANS: 3 sets of 20 reps

PUSHDOWNS (IF YOU HAVE BEEN USING A BAR, SWITCH TO ROPE OR VICE VERSA): 3 sets of 10 reps

MONDAY

REVERSE-BLUE-BAND DEADLIFTS (HANG BAND FROM TOP OF POWER CAGE): work up to max single

DUMBBELL ROWS: 2 sets of 10 reps, as heavy as possible

T-BAR ROWS: work up to heavy set of 6 reps

BARBELL SHRUGS: work up to heavy set of 10 reps in 3–4 sets

DUMBBELL CURLS: 3 sets of 10 reps

TUESDAY

STANDING PUSH-PRESS: work up to 5-rep max

CLOSE-GRIP BENCH: 3 work sets of 10, 8, and 6 reps, increasing weight each set

BARBELL, UPRIGHT ROWS: 3 work sets of 12, 10, and 8 reps, increasing weight each set

BENCH DIPS (PLACE PLATES IN LAP): 3 sets of 10 reps

WEEK FOUR: DELOAD WEEK

FRIDAY

SQUATS OFF PARALLEL BOX: 8 sets of doubles at 50% of max using only straight weight, wearing belt and briefs (if no briefs, wear suit bottoms)

WALKING LUNGES: 3 sets of 20 steps

PULL-THROUGHS: 3 sets of 20 reps

GLUTE/HAM RAISES OR HYPERS: 3 sets of 20 reps

CALF RAISES (ANY STYLE): 3 sets of 25 reps

SATURDAY

BENCH: 3 sets of 15 reps at 60% of max

LAT PULLS: work up to heavy set of six in a pyramid fashion over 3–4 sets

SEATED DUMBBELL POWER CLEANS: 3 sets of 20 reps

PUSHDOWNS (IF YOU HAVE BEEN USING A BAR, SWITCH TO ROPE OR VICE VERSA): 3 sets of 10 reps

MONDAY
(NO DEADLIFTS)
DUMBBELL ROWS: 2 sets of 10 reps, as heavy as possible
T-BAR ROWS: work up to heavy set of 6 reps
BARBELL SHRUGS: work up to heavy set of 10 reps in 3–4 sets
DUMBBELL CURLS: 3 sets of 10 reps

TUESDAY
SEATED DUMBBELL PRESSES (USE LIGHT WEIGHT): 2 sets of 10 reps
CLOSE-GRIP BENCH (USE LIGHT WEIGHT): 2 sets of 10 reps
BARBELL, UPRIGHT ROWS: 3 work sets of 12, 10, and 8 reps, increasing weight each set
BENCH DIPS (PLACE PLATES IN LAP): 3 sets of 10 reps (lighter than regular weeks)

FOURTH CYCLE
(CHANGED TO FIVE-DAY-A-WEEK SCHEDULE)

WEEK ONE

FRIDAY (WORK UP TO MAX SINGLE IN BRIEFS ONLY)
WALKING LUNGES: 3 sets of 20 steps
PULL-THROUGHS: 3 sets of 20 reps
GLUTE/HAM RAISES OR HYPERS: 3 sets of 20 reps
CALF RAISES (ANY STYLE): 3 sets of 25 reps

SATURDAY
FIVE-BOARD PRESSES: work up to 3-rep max

WEIGHTED DIPS (LEAN FORWARD TO EMPHASIZE CHEST): 3 sets of 10 reps

BARBELL INCLINE PRESSES: 3 sets of 10 reps

DUMBBELL FLIES: 2 sets of 10 reps

MONDAY

DEADS: standing on 4-inch platform, work up to 5-rep max

DUMBBELL ROWS: 2 sets of 10 reps, as heavy as possible

T-BAR ROWS: work up to heavy set of 6 reps

LAT PULLS: work up to heavy set of 6 in a pyramid fashion over 3–4 sets

CHINS: 3 sets to failure, at body weight

TUESDAY

SEATED DUMBBELL PRESSES: work up to 5-rep max

BARBELL, UPRIGHT ROWS: 3 work sets of 12, 10, and 8 reps, increasing weight each set

SHOULDER COMPLEX: do 20 front raises, 20 lateral raises, and 20 bent laterals; use dumbbells and perform one continuous set, moving immediately from one exercise to the next; rest then repeat 3 times

BARBELL SHRUGS: work up to heavy set of 10 reps in 3–4 sets

WEDNESDAY

CLOSE-GRIP BENCH: 3 work sets of 10, 8, and 6 reps, increasing weight each set

PUSHDOWNS: 3 sets of 10 reps

BENCH DIPS (PLACE PLATES IN LAP): 3 sets of 10 reps

BARBELL CURLS: 3 sets of 10 reps

SPIDER CURLS: 3 sets of 15 reps

DUMBBELL CONCENTRATION CURLS: 3 sets of 15 reps

WEEK TWO

FRIDAY (WORK UP TO MAX SINGLE IN BRIEFS AND SUIT BOTTOMS)
WALKING LUNGES: 3 sets of 20 steps
PULL-THROUGHS: 3 sets of 20 reps
GLUTE/HAM RAISES OR HYPERS: 3 sets of 20 reps
CALF RAISES (ANY STYLE): 3 sets of 25 reps

SATURDAY
FOUR-BOARD PRESSES: work up to 2-rep max
WEIGHTED DIPS (LEAN FORWARD TO EMPHASIZE CHEST): 3 sets of 10 reps
BARBELL INCLINE PRESSES: 3 sets of 10 reps
DUMBBELL FLIES: 2 sets of 10 reps

MONDAY
DEADS: standing on 2-inch platform, work up to 3-rep max
DUMBBELL ROWS: 2 sets of 10 reps, as heavy as possible
T-BAR ROWS: work up to heavy set of 6 reps
LAT PULLS: work up to heavy set of 6 in a pyramid fashion over 3–4 sets
CHINS: 3 sets to failure, at body weight

TUESDAY
SEATED PRESSES OFF PINS: in power rack, set height 1 inch above your head; work up to max triple
BARBELL, UPRIGHT ROWS: 3 work sets of 12, 10, and 8 reps, increasing weight each set
SHOULDER COMPLEX: do 20 front raises, 20 lateral raises, and 20 bent laterals; use dumbbells and perform one continuous set, moving immediately from one exercise to the next; rest then repeat 3 times
BARBELL SHRUGS: work up to heavy set of 10 reps in 3–4 sets

WEDNESDAY (PERFORM 3 SETS OF EACH SUPERSET)

SKULL CRUSHERS: 15 reps supersetted with 21s (perform skulls and then immediately stand up, grab same bar, and do a set of 21s [curls where you do 7 reps top half of the exercise, then 7 reps bottom half, then 7 reps full range, for total of 21 reps per set])
PUSHDOWNS: 15 reps supersetted with cable curls x20 reps
INCLINE DUMBBELL CURLS: for 10 reps supersetted, with incline dumbbell extensions x20 reps

WEEK THREE

FRIDAY (WORK UP TO MAX SINGLE IN FULL GEAR— BRIEFS, SUIT STRAPS-UP, WRAPS)

WALKING LUNGES: 3 sets of 20 steps
PULL-THROUGHS: 3 sets of 20 reps
GLUTE/HAM RAISES OR HYPERS: 3 sets of 20 reps
CALF RAISES (ANY STYLE): 3 sets of 25 reps

SATURDAY

THREE-BOARD PRESSES: work up to max single
WEIGHTED DIPS (LEAN FORWARD TO EMPHASIZE CHEST): 3 sets of 10 reps
BARBELL INCLINE PRESSES: 3 sets of 10 reps
DUMBBELL FLIES: 2 sets of 10 reps

MONDAY

DEADS FROM THE FLOOR: work up to max single
DUMBBELL ROWS: 2 sets of 10 reps, as heavy as possible
T-BAR ROWS: work up to heavy set of six reps
LAT PULLS: work up to heavy set of 6 in a pyramid fashion over 3–4 sets
CHINS: 3 sets to failure, using only body weight

TUESDAY

STANDING PUSH-PRESS: work up to max single

BARBELL UPRIGHT ROWS: 3 work sets of 12, 10, and 8 reps, increasing weight each set

SHOULDER COMPLEX: do 20 front raises, 20 lateral raises, and 20 bent laterals; use dumbbells and perform one continuous set, moving immediately from one exercise to the next; repeat 3 times

BARBELL SHRUGS: work up to heavy set of 10 reps in 3–4 sets

WEDNESDAY

CLOSE-GRIP BENCH: 3 work sets of 10, 8, and 6 reps, increasing weight each set

PUSHDOWNS: 3 sets of 10 reps

BENCH DIPS (PLACE PLATES IN LAP): 3 sets of 10 reps

BARBELL CURLS: 3 sets of 10 reps

SPIDER CURLS: 3 sets of 15 reps

DUMBBELL CONCENTRATION CURLS: 3 sets of 15 reps

WEEK FOUR: DELOAD WEEK

FRIDAY

SQUATS OFF PARALLEL BOX: 8 sets of doubles at 50% of max, using only straight weight, wearing belt and briefs

WALKING LUNGES: 3 sets of 20 steps

PULL-THROUGHS: 3 sets of 20 reps

GLUTE/HAM RAISES OR HYPERS: 3 sets of 20 reps

CALF RAISES (ANY STYLE): 3 sets of 25 reps

SATURDAY

BENCH: 3 sets of 15 reps at 60% of max

LAT PULLS: work up to heavy set of 6 in a pyramid fashion over 3–4 sets

BARBELL INCLINE PRESSES: 3 sets of 10 reps

DUMBBELL FLIES: 2 sets of 10 reps

MONDAY
(NO DEADLIFTS)

DUMBBELL ROWS: 2 sets of 10 reps, as heavy as possible

T-BAR ROWS: work up to heavy set of 6 reps

LAT PULLS: work up to heavy set of 6 in a pyramid fashion over 3–4 sets

CHINS: 3 sets to failure, using only body weight

TUESDAY

LIGHT SEATED DUMBBELL BELL PRESSES: 2 sets of 10 reps

SHOULDER COMPLEX: do 20 front raises, 20 lateral raises, and 20 bent laterals; use dumbbells and perform one continuous set, moving immediately from one exercise to the next; rest then repeat 3 times

WEDNESDAY (PERFORM 3 SETS OF EACH SUPERSET)

SKULL CRUSHERS: 15 reps supersetted with 21s (perform skulls and then immediately stand up, grab same bar, and do a set of 21s ([curls where you do 7 reps top half of the exercise, then 7 reps bottom half, then 7 reps full range, for total of 21 reps per set])

PUSHDOWNS: 15 reps supersetted with cable curls ×20 reps

INCLINE DUMBBELL CURLS: for 10 reps supersetted, with incline dumbbell extensions ×20 reps

TEN
POWERBUILDING

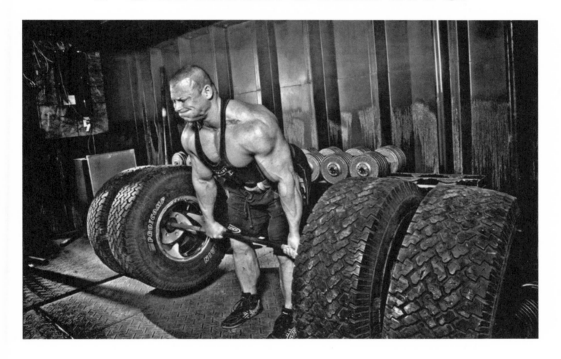

COMBINATION POWERLIFTING-BODYBUILDING PROGRAM

DAY ONE: CHEST

BENCH: warm up then follow weight progression listed at end of chapter

DIPS (WEIGHTED): pyramid up in weight sets of 10, 8, and 6; after last set, perform a triple drop set, reducing weight each set × 10 reps each

INCLINE BENCH: pyramid up in weight sets of 12, 10, 8 and triple drop set on last set

DUMBBELL INCLINE BENCH: pyramid up in weight sets of 12, 10, 8

DAY TWO: BACK

DEADLIFTS: warm up, then follow weight progression listed at end of chapter

LAT PULL-DOWNS: pyramid up in weight sets of 15, 12, 10, 8

T-BAR ROWS: pyramid up in weight sets of 12, 10, 8, 6

CHINS: 50 reps total in as many sets as it takes: rotate between 2–3 different grips

HEAVY DUMBBELL ROWS: 2 × 20, go as heavy on these as possible

BARBELL SHRUGS: 2 × 20, as heavy as possible

DAY THREE: SHOULDERS

STANDING MILITARY PRESS: warm up, then follow weight progression listed at end of chapter

SHOULDER COMPLEX: do 20 front raises, 20 lateral raises, and 20 bent laterals; use dumbbells and perform one continuous set, moving immediately from one exercise to the next; rest and then repeat 2 additional times.

DAY FOUR: ARMS

DUMBBELL OVERHEAD EXTENSION: pyramid up in weight sets of 12, 10, 8

PUSHDOWNS: pyramid up in weight sets of 12, 10, 8

BENCH DIPS: pyramid up in weight sets of 15, 12, 10

BARBELL CURLS: pyramid up in weight sets of 10, 8, 6

PREACHER CURLS: pyramid up in weight sets of 15, 12, 10

LYING CABLE CURLS: pyramid up in weight sets of 20, 15, 10 (do these from a high cable while lying on your back on a bench; curl the EZ-curl handle to your forehead)

DAY FIVE: LEGS

SQUATS: warm up, then follow weight progression listed at end of chapter

FRONT SQUATS: 2×20

WALKING LUNGES: 2×30 steps

LYING LEG CURLS: 3×10

SEATED LEG CURLS: 3×20

ANY TYPE OF CALF RAISE: 3×25

WEIGHT PROGRESSION FOR SQUATS, BENCH, MILITARY PRESSES, AND DEADLIFTS

WEEK 1	5 x 10 x 60%; no deads (5 sets of 10 reps at 60%)
WEEK 2	5 x 8 x 65%
WEEK 3	5 x 5 x 70%
WEEK 4	5 x 3 x 75%
WEEK 5	5 x 10 x 60%; no deads
WEEK 6	5 x 8 x 70%
WEEK 7	5 x 5 x 75%
WEEK 8	5 x 3 x 80%
WEEK 9	5 x 10 x 60%; no deads
WEEK 10	4 x 8 x 75%
WEEK 11	4 x 5 x 80%
WEEK 12	4 x 3 x 85%
WEEK 13	5 x 10 x 60%; no deads
WEEK 14	3 x 8 x 80%
WEEK 15	3 x 5 x 85%
WEEK 16	3 x 3 x 90%
WEEK 17	find new maxes on squat, bench, and deads

ELEVEN
DOUBLE-SPLIT
STRENGTH PROGRAM

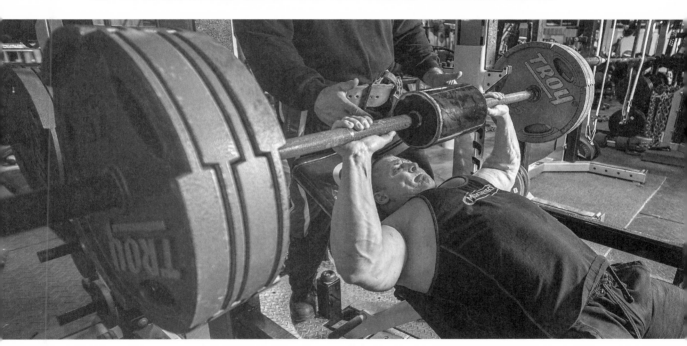

This training program is designed around a four-day training week. It features a split that alternates the assistance work every other week. The main compound lifts, however, are trained following a weekly progression over a sixteen-week training cycle. It is a challenging program, but, followed to the letter, it will yield impressive gains in strength and size. Before starting this program, you will need to take true maxes on your squat, bench, deadlifts, and standing military presses. It is important that those numbers are accurate and that you never over-estimate your maxes, which will lead to overtraining and a lack of progress. This program is built around basic compound movements, which will yield the greatest gains in size and strength when trained properly.

TRAINING WEEK A (WEEKS 1, 3, 5, 7, 9, 11, 13, 15)

DAY ONE: CHEST AND TRICEPS

BENCH: warm up, then follow weight progression detailed at the end of the chapter.

INCLINE BARBELL PRESSES: at 15-to-25-degree angle, pyramid up in weight for sets of 10, 8, 6 reps

DUMBBELL TWIST PRESSES: Perform these by starting just as you would for a traditional dumbbell bench press. As you press the weight up, however, twist your wrists so that, at the top of the movement, your palms are supinated like a reverse-grip bench press. Then touch the ends of the dumbbells together. Start light and work up in small increments for sets of 10 reps until you can no longer fully rotate the dumbbells at the top. This is much harder than a regular dumbbell bench press. At least 4 of these sets should be work sets.

V-BAR PUSHDOWNS: 4 sets of 15 reps (only 45-second rest between sets)

SKULL CRUSHERS: 4 sets of 15 reps (only 45-second rest between sets)

DAY TWO: BACK AND BICEPS

DEADLIFTS: warm up, then follow weight progression detailed at the end of the chapter.

CHINS: 50 reps total in as many sets as it takes; rotate between 2–3 different grips (use a chin-assistance machine if you can't do at least 10 reps on your own)

KROC ROWS: 2 warm-up sets, then 1×20; go as heavy on these as possible (no straps)

CHEST-SUPPORTED ROWS: pyramid up in weight for sets of 10, 8, 6 reps

BARBELL CURLS: (straight bar) 4 sets of 15 reps (only 45-second rest between sets)

DUMBBELL INCLINE CURLS: 4 sets of 15 reps (only 45-second rest between sets)

DAY THREE
Rest on day three.

DAY FOUR: SHOULDERS
STANDING MILITARY PRESS: warm up, then follow weight progression detailed at the end of the chapter.

SEATED DUMBBELL POWER CLEANS: pyramid up in weight for sets of 15, 12, 10 reps

LEANING DUMBBELL LATERAL RAISES: 3 sets of 15 reps

BENT LATERAL RAISES: pyramid up in weight for sets of 15, 12, 10 reps

BARBELL SHRUGS: pyramid up in weight for sets of 15, 12, 10 reps

DAY FIVE: LEGS
SQUATS: warm up, then follow weight progression detailed at the end of the chapter.

WALKING LUNGES: 2×30 steps (you can hold dumbbells, use chains around your neck, or carry a barbell on your shoulders in the standard back-squat position)

LEG EXTENSION: pyramid up in weight for sets of 15, 12, 10 reps

STIFF-LEGGED DEADLIFTS WITH DUMBBELLS: pyramid up in weight for sets of 10, 8, 6 reps

LYING LEG CURLS: pyramid up in weight for sets of 15, 12, 10 reps

CALF TRISET: After warming up, start with calf raises on the leg press machine and use a weight that allows 20 reps. Get off the leg press and immediately start doing standing calf raises off an elevated platform with just your body weight for 25 reps. Then go immediately to the seated calf machine and do another 20 reps. Repeat this three times, and you're done for the day. Rest for 2–3 minutes between sets.

DAYS SIX AND SEVEN
Rest on these days.

TRAINING WEEK B (WEEKS 2, 4, 6, 8, 10, 12, 14, 16)

DAY ONE: CHEST AND TRICEPS
BENCH: warm up, then follow weight progression detailed at the end of the chapter.

INCLINE DUMBBELL PRESSES: at 15-to-25-degree angle, do 4 sets of 10 reps

DIPS: 3 sets to failure with body weight

ROPE PUSHDOWNS: 4 sets of 15 reps (only 45-second rest between sets)

BENCH DIPS: put plates in your lap to add resistance and do 4 sets of 15 reps (only 45-second rest between sets)

DAY TWO: BACK AND BICEPS
DEADLIFTS: warm up, then follow weight progression detailed at the end of the chapter.

HEAVY DUMBBELL ROWS: do 2 warm-up sets, then 1×20; go as heavy on these as possible (use straps)

LAT PULL-DOWNS: using wide overhand grip, do 4 sets of 15 reps

T-BAR ROWS: pyramid up, adding a plate each set (45 or 25 pounds, depending on your strength level) until you cannot get 10 reps (should take at least 4–5 sets)

SEATED BARBELL CURLS: 4 sets of 15 reps (only 45-second rest between sets)

DUMBBELL SPIDER CURLS: 4 sets of 15 reps (only 45-second rest between sets)

DAY THREE

Rest on day three.

DAY FOUR: SHOULDERS

STANDING MILITARY PRESS: warm up, then follow weight progression detailed at the end of the chapter.

SHOULDER COMPLEX: do 20 front raises, 20 lateral raises, and 20 bent laterals; use dumbbells and perform one continuous set, moving immediately from one exercise to the next without rest; rest and then repeat 3 times

REAR DELT LATERALS ON MACHINE: 3 sets of 20 reps

DUMBBELL SHRUGS: work up to max set of 10 reps, then 3×10 reps; go as heavy as possible

DAY FIVE: LEGS

SQUATS: warm up, then follow weight progression detailed at the end of the chapter.

LEG PRESS: This is a technique that I call an up-and-down set. Make no mistake: this will be brutal. First, warm up by working up to a weight that is about 60% of your 10-rep max, and then do just one all-out up-and-down set. Trust me: one of these will be enough. This is how it works: perform 5 reps with the 60% and then hold the weight at lockout (the weight is never racked until all the sets are done) and have your training partners add a plate to each side and do another 5 reps; then hold it at lockout as they add another plate to each side. Keep doing 5 reps at each weight and going up until you can barely get 5 reps (this should take at least 4–5 sets). Even though your legs will be on fire, you're only halfway done. Next have your partners start stripping weights a plate at a time and do 5 reps at each weight until you get back down to where you started. Your legs should be burning like never before. You should be able to perform around 10 sets total with about 50 total reps.

BULGARIAN SPLIT SQUATS: 3 sets of 12 reps on each leg

STIFF-LEGGED DEADS: with dumbbells, do 4 sets of 10 reps

SEATED LEG CURLS: 3 sets of 20 reps

CALF TRISET: After warming up a bit, start with calf raises on the leg press machine and use a weight that allows 20 reps. Get off the leg press and immediately start doing standing calf raises off an elevated platform with just your body weight for 25 reps. Then go immediately to the seated calf machine and do another 20 reps. Repeat this three times, and you're done for the day. Rest 2–3 minutes between sets.

DAYS SIX AND SEVEN

Rest on these days.

WEIGHT PROGRESSION FOR SQUATS, BENCH, MILITARY PRESSES, AND DEADLIFTS

WEEK 1	5 x 10 x 60% (5 sets of 10 reps at 60%); no deadlifts
WEEK 2	5 x 8 x 65%
WEEK 3	5 x 5 x 70%
WEEK 4	5 x 3 x 75%
WEEK 5	5 x 10 x 60%; no deadlifts
WEEK 6	5 x 8 x 70%
WEEK 7	5 x 5 x 75%
WEEK 8	5 x 3 x 80%
WEEK 9	5 x 10 x 60%; no deadlifts

WEEK 10	4 x 8 x 75%
WEEK 11	4 x 5 x 80%
WEEK 12	4 x 3 x 85%
WEEK 13	5 x 10 x 60%; no deadlifts
WEEK 14	3 x 8 x 80%
WEEK 15	3 x 5 x 85%
WEEK 16	3 x 3 x 90%

TWELVE
KROC TRIPLE-THREAT
TRAINING PROGRAM

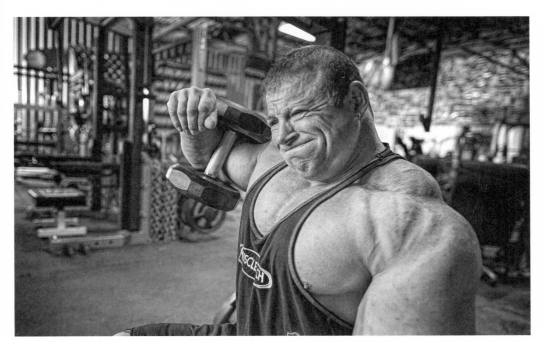

This is a bodybuilding-style training program designed for advanced lifters who have plateaued and are looking for something to shock their body into additional size and strength gains. It is very challenging and will require proper nutritional support and sufficient rest in order to reap the full benefits and avoid overtraining. It is comprised of three distinct phases that are each performed for one week, and then a fourth week (not included in the program) should be a light, easy recovery-style training week before starting the three phases again.

PHASE ONE: HEAVY

LEGS
REVERSE BAND SQUATS: work up to heavy triple in 4–5 sets
LEG PRESS: work up to heavy set of 6 reps in 4–5 sets
PULL-THROUGHS: 2 sets of 20 reps
BAND LEG CURLS: 4 sets of 20 reps

CHEST
REVERSE BAND BENCH: work up to heavy triple in 4–5 sets
DUMBBELL INCLINE PRESS: work up to heavy set of 6 reps in 3–4 sets
DIPS: work up to heavy set of 6 reps in 3–4 sets

BACK
DEADS: work up to heavy single
KROC ROWS: with straps, work up to a max set of 10 reps
WEIGHTED CHINS: work up to heavy set of 6 reps in 3–4 sets
T-BAR ROWS: work up to heavy set of 6 reps in 3–4 sets

SHOULDERS
MILITARY PRESSES: work up to heavy triple in 4–5 sets
PARTIAL-RANGE CHEAT LATERALS: work up to heavy set of 6 reps in 3–4 sets
SEATED DUMBBELL POWER CLEANS: work up to heavy set of 10 reps in 3–4 sets
BENT LATERALS: work up to heavy set of 6 reps in 3–4 sets
FARMER'S-WALK SHRUGS: 2 sets of 20 reps

ARMS

BARBELL CURLS: work up to heavy set of 6 reps in 3–4 sets

SEATED DUMBBELL CURLS: work up to heavy set of 6 reps in 3–4 sets

DUMBBELL SCOTT CURLS: work up to heavy set of 6 reps in 3–4 sets

CHAIN CLOSE-GRIP BENCH: work up to heavy set of 6 reps in 3–4 sets

CHAIN SKULL CRUSHERS: work up to heavy set of 6 reps in 3–4 sets

BENCH DIPS: work up to heavy set of 6 reps in 3–4 sets

PHASE TWO: INTENSITY

LEGS

SSB SQUATS WITH CHAINS: work up to max set of 10 reps, then drop chains and rep until failure

LEG PRESS: work up to heavy set of 10 reps, then perform four drop sets to equal 50 total reps

STIFF-LEGGED DEADS: work up to heavy set of 20, then perform a double drop set

BACK RAISES/HYPERS WITH BANDS (START WITH 3 LIGHT BANDS): triple drop set of 10 reps each

CHEST

BENCH: work up to heavy set of 5 reps in 4–5 sets but with 4–5 forced reps on every set

INCLINES: work up to heavy set of 5 reps in 4–5 sets but with 4–5 forced reps on every set

DIPS: work up to heavy set of 10 reps, then triple drop for 40 total reps

BACK

KROC ROWS: without straps, work up to a max set of 20–30 reps

WEIGHTED CHINS: work up to heavy set of 8 reps, then triple drop

T-BAR ROWS: work up to heavy set of 10 reps, then triple drop

LAT PULLS: work up to heavy set of 10 reps, then triple drop

SHOULDERS

PLATE RAISES: work up to heavy set of 10 reps, then triple drop

SHOULDER COMPLEX TRISET: do 20 seated dumbbell front raises, 20 seated dumbbell lateral raises, and 20 seated bent laterals, performed consecutively without rest between exercises; rest and repeat 2 times

BAND PULL-APARTS: triple drop set of 20 reps each; start with light and miniband

ARMS

EZ-BAR CURLS: work up to heavy set of 10 reps then quadruple drop set for a total of 50 reps

CABLE CURLS: work up to heavy set of 10 reps then quadruple drop set for a total of 50 reps

DUMBBELL CONCENTRATION CURLS: one set, trading arms back and forth without rest; do 20, 15, 10, 5 reps

ROPE PUSHDOWNS: work up to heavy set of 10 reps then quadruple drop set for a total of 50 reps

BENCH DIPS: heavy set of 10 reps then quadruple drop set for a total of 50 reps

DUMBBELL KICKBACKS: one set, trading arms back and forth without rest; do 20, 15, 10, 5 reps

PHASE THREE: HIGH VOLUME

LEGS

SAFETY-SQUAT-BAR SQUATS: work up to heavy set of 10 reps for 4 sets

LEG PRESS: work up to heavy set of 10 reps for 4 sets

HACK SQUATS: 4 sets of 25 reps
LOG LUNGES: 4 sets of 20 steps
PULL-THROUGHS: 4 sets of 25 reps
BAND LEG CURLS: 4 sets of 25 reps

CHEST

BENCH: work up to heavy set of 8 reps for 4 sets
INCLINES: work up to heavy set of 8 reps for 4 sets
DUMBBELL BENCH PRESS: work up to heavy set of 8 reps for 4 sets
DUMBBELL INCLINE PRESS: work up to heavy set of 6 reps in 3–4 sets
DIPS: work up to heavy set of 8 reps for 4 sets

BACK

WEIGHTED CHINS: work up to heavy set of 8 reps for 4 sets
T-BAR ROWS: work up to heavy set of 8 reps for 4 sets
LAT PULLS: work up to heavy set of 8 reps for 4 sets
SEATED CABLE ROWS, WIDE GRIP: work up to heavy set of 8 reps for 4 sets
CLOSE-GRIP LAT PULL-DOWNS: work up to heavy set of 8 reps for 4 sets

SHOULDERS

SEATED DUMBBELL PRESSES: work up to heavy set of 8 reps for 4 sets
UPRIGHT ROWS: work up to heavy set of 8 reps for 4 sets
SEATED LATERAL RAISES: work up to heavy set of 8 reps for 4 sets
BENT LATERALS: work up to heavy set of 8 reps for 4 sets
BARBELL SHRUGS: work up to heavy set of 8 reps for 4 sets

ARMS

EZ-BAR CURLS: work up to heavy set of 8 reps for 4 sets
LYING CABLE CURLS: work up to 12 reps for 4 sets
DUMBBELL SCOTT CURLS: work up to heavy set of 8 reps for 4 sets

DUMBBELL SPIDER CURLS: work up to heavy set of 15 reps for 4 sets
CHAIN CLOSE-GRIP BENCH: work up to heavy set of 8 reps for 4 sets
CHAIN SKULL CRUSHERS: work up to heavy set of 8 reps for 4 sets
PUSHDOWNS: work up to heavy set of 8 reps for 4 sets
DUMBBELL KICKBACKS: work up to 15 reps for 4 sets

THIRTEEN
PYRAMID, PLUS A PUMP ARM-TRAINING

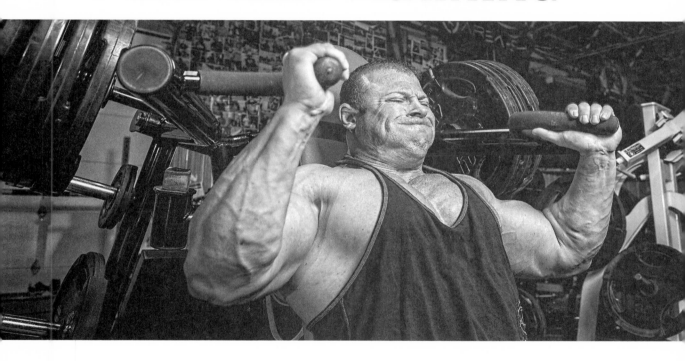

This arm-training program combines basic movements with a pyramid-style rep scheme and adds a twist. On the last set of each exercise, perform a triple drop set by decreasing the weight by approximately 20–25% and, without rest, immediately grind out more reps until you reach failure again. Perform this drop three times without rest on the last set of each exercise. This will force a ton of blood into your arms, stretching the fascia and allowing room for new muscle growth to occur.

THE TRAINING PROGRAM

CLOSE-GRIP BENCH PRESSES: pyramid up in weight for sets of 10, 8, 6, then triple drop set on last set

PUSHDOWNS: pyramid up in weight for sets of 15, 12, 10, then triple drop set on last set

SKULL CRUSHERS: pyramid up in weight for sets of 15, 12, 10, then triple drop set on last set

BENCH DIPS: 100 total reps in 4 or more sets (if you can do this in fewer than four sets, add more weight)

BARBELL CURLS: pyramid up in weight for sets of 20, 15, 10, then triple drop set on last set

PREACHER CURLS: pyramid up in weight for sets of 20, 15, 10, then triple drop set on last set

DUMBBELL SPIDER CURLS: pyramid up in weight for sets of 20, 15, 10, then triple drop set on last set

LYING CABLE CURLS: lie flat on your back on a bench, feet facing high-cable-pulley machine; using a short EZ-curl attachment, curl the bar to your forehead; do 20, 15, 10 and then triple drop set on last set

THE EXERCISES

CLOSE-GRIP BENCH: This is a basic mass-building movement for the triceps that will allow you to handle relatively heavy weights. As the name implies, you want to perform close-grip bench presses with a relatively narrow grip, where your hands are just inside your shoulder width. At the bottom of the movement, when the bar is at your chest, your hands should be just outside your torso. The key here is to concentrate on tucking your elbows into your sides as hard as possible during the eccentric portion of the movement to shift the focus onto the triceps. You will be touching the bar low on your chest, usually just below your pecs, depending on your individual leverages.

You should also attempt to keep the elbows tucked in as your press the weight back up.

BENCH DIPS: Set up two benches parallel to each other. They should be just far enough apart so that when you have your feet up on one bench with your legs straight, there is room for you to descend in front of the opposite bench without scraping your back against it. Position your hands just outside shoulder width, behind you and pronated so that your palms are on the bench. The movement is very similar to a conventional dip, but, by moving the hand position farther to the rear, it largely takes your pecs out of the movement, and your triceps become the primary mover. Descend in between the benches until your upper arms are parallel to the floor. To add resistance, have a training partner load weight plates onto your lap.

STRAIGHT BARBELL CURLS: These are one of the primary means to build mass and strength for the biceps. Performing them with a straight barbell instead of an EZ-curl bar further supinates the grip and forces the biceps to contract to a greater degree at the top of the movement. Your grip should typically be shoulder width or just slightly farther apart, but the grip width can be varied to attack the biceps from slightly different angles. One effective technique for barbell curls is to perform as many reps as possible in strict form; then, once you reach muscular failure, use a moderate amount of body English to grind out several more reps. This should be done to make the exercise harder, not easier. If you find yourself cheating up the reps throughout the entire set, then you need to reduce the weight and check your ego.

DUMBBELL SPIDER CURLS: By allowing you to get a really hard contraction at the top of the movement, these stand in contrast to most curling movements, where the amount of stress on the biceps is actually reduced at the top of the curl. Perform them by lying facedown on an incline bench set at about 45 degrees or slightly less. While lying on the bench, grab the dumbbells from the floor and curl them all the way up while fully supinating your grip, thus forcing the biceps to contract hard at the completion of the movement. The forward lean of the exercise keeps the stress on the muscle throughout the range of motion and never allows the biceps to rest. These are typically most effective when performed for higher rep ranges (10–20) and with a moderate amount of weight.

FOURTEEN
DETAILED BODY-BUILDING PROGRAM

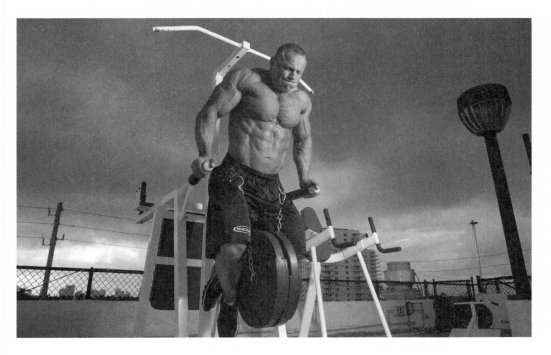

With bodybuilding programs, our priorities are gaining muscle size, shape, and balance; strength gains are a goal only because they provide a means to increase muscle hypertrophy. This program focuses on using overall volume, short rest periods, specific angles, and intensity techniques to induce as much muscle growth as possible. Working with John Meadows over the last couple of years has greatly influenced my philosophy concerning bodybuilding training, and those of you who are

107

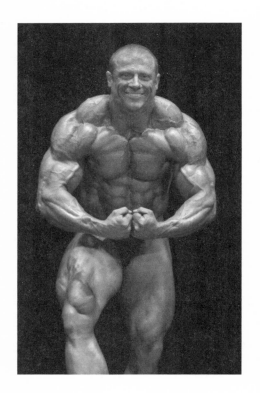

familiar with John and his Mountain Dog training may recognize his influence on the design and style of my programming for bodybuilding. John possesses one of the greatest minds in the sport of bodybuilding and is someone for whom I have a great deal of respect and admiration. I have learned a lot from John and consider him to be one of my mentors.

The following sample program is based on a five-day training week and breaks the individual training session down into five distinct days, with one each dedicated to chest, back, shoulders, arms, and legs. The sessions can be performed on any day of the week, and the two nontraining days placed anywhere that suits your weekly schedule, but the days must remain in the specific order described below since the program is designed to give each individual muscle group sufficient recovery time before being worked hard again.

WEEK ONE

DAY ONE: CHEST

DUMBBELL TWIST PRESSES: Perform these by starting just as you would for a traditional dumbbell bench press. As you press the weight up, however, twist your wrists so that, at the top of the movement, your palms are supinated like a reverse-grip bench press. Then, touch the ends of the dumbbells together. Start light and work up in small increments for sets of 10 reps until you can no longer fully rotate the dumbbells at the top. This is much harder than a regular dumbbell bench press. At least 4 of these sets should be work sets. Rest 2–3 minutes between sets.

INCLINE BARBELL PRESSES: Use a low incline that is at an angle of approximately 15–25 degrees. Work up in 2–3 sets to a fairly tough set of 5 reps and stay there for 5 sets of 5 reps. Rest 2–3 minutes between sets.

LADDER PUSH-UPS: You can put a bar inside a power cage for these, setting pins at three different heights. Or, use a Smith machine if you have access to one. The first setting should be as low to the ground as possible. Pump out as many reps as possible, but stop 2–4 reps short of failure. Then, move the bar up six to ten inches and pump out as many as possible, but this time go to failure. Next, move the bar up another 6–10 inches and go again until failure. Your chest should be totally engorged with blood at this point. If you can do more than 25 reps on the first set, add resistance by having your training partners drape chains across your back in an X. Perform 3 sets, resting 2–3 minutes between sets.

DAY TWO: BACK

KROC ROWS: Work up in 3 to 4 sets of 10 reps to one really heavy all-out, high-rep set of at least 20 reps per arm. If you get more than 25 reps, next time add more weight.

CHINS: Perform a total of 100 reps in as many sets as it takes to get there. Vary the hand placement on each set. Start with a wide overhand grip; then use a medium, neutral grip; and finish with a close grip, using a V bar. Then start over with the wide grip. If you can't get at least 10 reps per set, use a chin-assistance machine or bands to help you get the desired number of reps. Try to take the biceps out of the movement as much as possible and focus on using your lats throughout the movement. Rest 2–3 minutes between sets.

T-BAR ROWS: Use a V bar with a barbell in a landmine-type device or with the end of the barbell shoved in a corner. Work up a 45 pound plate (or 25-pound plate at a time, depending on your strength level) at 10 reps per set until you can no longer get 10 reps. At least 4 of these should be work sets. Rest 2–3 minutes between sets.

BARBELL SHRUGS: Use a double-over hand grip and just focus on moving your shoulders up and down (after warming up) with as much weight as possible for 3 sets of 20 reps.

DAY THREE: SHOULDERS

SEATED CHAIN LATERAL RAISES: Clip D handles to chains and, after 1–2 warm-ups, perform 3 sets of 20 reps with a smooth and controlled tempo. On the last rep, hold the weight at lockout for as long as possible. Concentrate on using your medial delts to move the weight, and avoid shrugging your shoulders up or back to keep the traps out of the movement as much as possible. Rest 2–3 minutes between sets.

DUMBBELL BENT LATERALS: Sit on the end of a flat bench and bend forward far enough to allow the dumbbells to touch under your legs at the bottom of the movement. Perform 3 sets of 20 reps. Again, focus on using the rear delts and try to engage the traps as little as possible. Rest 2–3 minutes between sets.

SEATED DUMBBELL PRESSES: Work up slowly in sets of 6 reps until you reach your max set of 6. At least 4 of these should feel like work sets. Rest 2–3 minutes between sets.

DUMBBELL SHRUGS: Do 2–3 warm-up sets and then perform 4 sets of 25 reps with heavy dumbbells. Use straps here so that your grip isn't the limiting factor and just shrug the weight straight up and down with the greatest range of motion possible.

DAY FOUR: ARMS

DOWN-THE-RACK BARBELL CURLS: Warm up, then start with a weight that you can get 10 reps with but still have 2–3 reps in the tank. As soon as you get to 10, either strip some weight (loading all 10-pound or 5-pound plates on a barbell works well) or grab a barbell that is approximately 10–20% lighter and do another 10 reps. Then drop again and do 10 reps at each drop for a total of 4 drops, which equals 5 sets for a total of 50 reps. Your arms should be totally filled with blood from just one long drop set of this.

DUMBBELL CURLS: Keep your palm supinated at all times (palm up) and perform all reps with one arm, then switch to the other arm. Perform 10 reps per set.

SUPERSETTED WITH:

DUMBBELL HAMMER CURLS: Do these straight up and down like a regular curl, not across the body. Again, perform all reps with one arm, then switch to the other arm. Perform 10 reps per set.

Perform 4 sets of each superset for 8 sets total between the two exercises. Rest 2–3 minutes between each superset.

EZ-BAR PREACHER REVERSE CURLS: Perform 10 reps per set. Start this superset with your palms facing down in a reverse-curl fashion.

SUPERSETTED WITH:

EZ-BAR PREACHER CURLS: Reverse your grip so that your palms face up and keep going. Perform 10 reps per set.

Perform 4 sets of each superset for 8 sets total between the two exercises. Rest 2–3 minutes between each superset.

ROPE PUSHDOWNS: Get full extension and push the rope apart at the bottom. Perform 15 reps per set.

SUPERSETTED WITH:

OVERHEAD ROPE EXTENSIONS: Simply turn around after finishing the pushdowns and do another 15 reps, leaning away from the machine and extend the rope overhead. It is okay to lighten the weight some if necessary to complete all the reps.

Perform 4 sets of each superset for 8 sets total between the two exercises. Rest 2–3 minutes between each superset.

OVERHEAD DUMBBELL EXTENSIONS: Get full extension at the top and a decent stretch at the bottom. Perform 15 reps per set.

SUPERSETTED WITH:

BENCH DIPS: Set up two benches of the same height and perform dips in between them. Have your partner place plates in your lap to add resistance. Perform 20 reps per set.

Perform 4 sets of each superset for 8 sets total between the two exercises. Rest 2–3 minutes between each superset.

SKULL-CRUSHER DROP SET: Your elbows should be warmed up well by now, so do one warm-up set and then start with a weight that you can get 12–15 reps with, but only do 10. As soon as you get to 10, strip approximately 10–20% of the weight (loading all 10-pound or 5-pound plates on the barbell works well) and do another 10 reps. Then drop again and do 10 reps at each drop for a total of 4 drops, which equals 5 sets for a total of 50 reps. Your arms should be totally filled with blood from just one long drop set of this.

DAY FIVE: LEGS

CHAIN SQUATS: Warm up and work up to a weight that is 60% of what you can do for a max set of 6 reps. Then start adding a chain per side for each set of 6 reps until you can no longer get 6 reps. This should take 3–5 sets. Rest 2–3 minutes between sets.

LEG PRESS: Perform what I call an up-and-down set. This will be brutal. First work up to a weight that is about 60% of your 10-rep max, and then do one all-out up-and-down set. Trust me: one of these will be enough. This is how it works: perform 5 reps with the 60% and then hold the weight at lockout (the weight is never racked until all the sets are done) and have your training partners add a plate to each side and do another 5 reps; then hold it at lockout as they add another plate to each side. Keep doing 5 reps at each weight and going up until you can barely get 5 reps (this should take at least 4–5 sets). Even though your legs will be on fire, you're only halfway done. Next have your partners start stripping weights a plate at a time and do 5 reps at each weight until you get back down to where you started. Your legs should be burning like never before. You should be able to perform around 10 sets total with about 50 total reps.

CHAIN LUNGES: Throw the appropriate amount of chains around your neck and take 30 steps (15 reps with each leg), touching your knee to the ground on each step. Do this for 4 sets of 30 steps. Rest 2–3 minutes between sets.

BARBELL STIFF-LEGGED DEADS: Use 25-pound plates for these or stand on a 4-inch platform to increase the range of motion. Keep your chest up and lower back arched and concentrate on using your hams to move the weight. Keep a slight bend in your knees throughout the movement. Do not rest the weight on the floor during the set to keep tension on the muscles at all times. Work up to a hard set of 10 reps and then stay there for 4 sets of 10 reps. Rest 2–3 minutes between sets.

SEATED LEG CURLS: work up to 3 sets of 10 reps. But on the last set

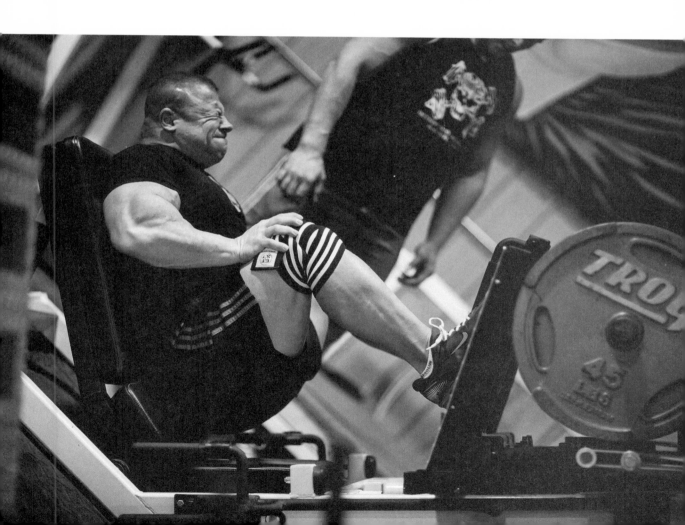

do a triple drop set, hitting 10 reps at each weight for a total of 40 reps on the last set. If you don't have a machine, use bands while sitting on a bench with the bands attached to a sturdy structure about 3–4 feet away. Perform the drop set by using progressively lighter bands. Rest 2–3 minutes between sets.

CALF TRISET: After warming up a bit, start with calf raises on the leg-press machine and use a weight that allows 20 reps. Get off the leg press and immediately start doing standing calf raises off an elevated platform with just your body weight for 25 reps. Then go immediately to the seated calf machine and do another 20 reps. Repeat this three times, and you're done for the day. Rest 2–3 minutes between sets.

WEEK TWO

DAY ONE: CHEST

REVERSE-BAND BENCH PRESS: Use medium to heavy bands that are hung from the top of a power rack. Warm up and work up to a heavy set of 5 reps, then stay there for 5 sets of 5 reps. Rest 2–3 minutes between sets.

INCLINE DUMBBELL PRESSES: Use a low incline that is at an angle of approximately 15–25 degrees. Work up in 2–3 sets to a fairly tough set of 10 reps and stay there for 4 sets of 10 reps. Rest 2–3 minutes between sets.

WEIGHTED DIPS: Lean forward on these and focus on using your chest, not your triceps, to move the weight. Avoid fully locking out to keep the tension on the chest. Work up to a set of 10 reps with as much weight as possible. Stay there for 3 sets of 10 reps, but on the last set do a triple drop set. So do your 10 reps and then drop enough weight to allow you to do 10 more reps with effort. Next drop all the weight and do 10 more reps with just your body weight. Rest 2–3 minutes between sets.

DAY TWO: BACK

ONE-ARM BARBELL ROWS: If you have a Meadows row handle, use it for these. If not, just grasp the barbell at the very end, near the inside collar. Place the other end of the barbell in a landmine apparatus or shove it into a corner. Load just the one end of the barbell and use 25-pound or 10-pound plates on these to allow for a full range of motion. Work up to a hard set of 10 reps, then stay there for 4 sets. Rest 2–3 minutes between sets.

WIDE-OVERHAND-GRIP LAT PULL-DOWNS: Try to take the biceps out of the movement as much as possible and focus on using your lats throughout the movement. Work up to a hard set of 10 reps, then stay there for 4 sets. Rest 2–3 minutes between sets.

CHEST-SUPPORTED ROWS: Work up to a heavy set of 8 reps and then stay there for 4 sets. Rest 2–3 minutes between sets.

DUMBBELL SHRUGS: Use straps and the heaviest dumbbells possible and then just focus on moving your shoulders up and down (after warming up) with as much weight as possible for 3 sets of 20 reps. Rest 2–3 minutes between sets.

BANDED HYPEREXTENSIONS: Use a shortened light band and put it over your head and around your neck. Perform 30 sets of 20 reps, but make the last set a drop set by doing your 20 reps and then dropping the band and going until failure. Rest 2–3 minutes between sets.

DAY THREE: SHOULDERS

LEANING LATERAL RAISES: Grab onto a sturdy structure with one hand and hold the dumbbell in the other. Keeping your feet together and close to the structure, lean away from it until your arm is straight. This will make the movement very strict and hit the medial delt hard. After 1–2 warm-ups, perform 3 sets of 20 reps with a smooth and controlled tempo. Rest 2–3 minutes between sets.

BAND PULL-APARTS: Perform 4 sets of 25 reps. Focus on using the rear delts and try to engage the traps as little as possible. Rest 2–3 minutes between sets.

STANDING MILITARY PRESSES: Work up slowly in sets of 6 reps until you reach your max set of 6. At least 4 of these should feel like work sets. Rest 2–3 minutes between sets.

BARBELL SHRUGS: Perform 2–3 feeder sets and then do 5 sets of 10 reps, as heavy as possible. Just shrug the weight straight up and down since there is no reason to roll your shoulders or move them in a horizontal plane during the movement.

DAY FOUR: ARMS

DOWN-THE-RACK DUMBBELL CURLS: Curl these with both arms at the same time. Warm up and then start with a weight that you can get 10 reps with but still have 2–3 reps in the tank. As soon as you get to 10, put those dumbbells down and grab a pair that's 10–20 pounds lighter and do another 10 reps. Then keep doing drops and do 10 reps at each drop for a total of 4 drops, which equals 5 sets for a total of 50 reps. Your arms should be totally filled with blood from just one long drop set of this.

V-BAR PUSHDOWN DROP SET: Using the same method as above, warm up and then complete a set of 10 reps with a weight that, at most, would allow you to do 12–13 reps. Then immediately move the pin up a couple holes and do 10 more reps. Keep doing this for a total of 5 drop sets for a total of 50 reps.

CABLE CURLS: Use a curl-bar attachment on the low pulley. Use a weight that you can get about 20 reps with, but only do 15 reps. Do this for 5 sets. The kicker is that you'll only be resting for 45 seconds between sets. Your arms will swell huge from the high volume and short rest periods.

LYING DUMBBELL EXTENSIONS: Lie flat on your back and perform a skull-crusher-type movement with dumbbells, except keep your palms facing each other and bring the dumbbells down to your shoulders instead of your forehead before firing them back up. Perform 5 sets of 10 reps with only 45 seconds' rest between sets.

REVERSE CURLS WITH EZ-CURL BAR: Use a weight that you can get about 20 reps with, but only do 15 reps. Do this for 5 sets. Again, the kicker is that you'll only be resting for 45 seconds between sets. Your biceps and forearms will swell huge from the high volume and short rest periods.

SKULL CRUSHERS ON AN INCLINE BENCH: Use an EZ-curl bar for these and perform 5 sets of 10 reps with only 45 seconds' rest between sets.

DAY FIVE: LEGS

REVERSE BAND SQUATS: Use medium or heavy bands suspended from the top of the squat rack for these. Warm up and then work up to a max set of 6 reps. This should take 3–5 work sets, not counting warm-up sets. Rest 2–3 minutes between sets.

LEG PRESS: Work up to a fairly difficult set of 10 reps—not an absolute max, but something you have to work for. Stay at that weight, and on your next set dig down and get 20 reps. Stay at that weight again, but this time give it everything you've got and find a way to get 30 reps without racking the weight. You can rest at lockout and use your hands to push on your knees—whatever it takes—but find a way to get all 30 reps. Rest 3–5 minutes between sets.

BULGARIAN SPLIT SQUATS: Put one foot up on a bench behind you with the other foot out front. Squat down on your front leg so that you're in a lunge-type position in the bottom and then push back up with your front leg. Perform 3 sets of 12 reps with each leg. Rest 2–3 minutes between sets.

DUMBBELL STIFF-LEGGED DEADS: Keep your chest up and lower back arched and concentrate on using your hams to move the weight. Keep a slight bend in your knees throughout the movement. Do not rest the weight on the floor during the set; keep tension on the muscles at all times. Work up to a hard set of 10 reps and then stay there for 4 sets of 10 reps. Rest 2–3 minutes between sets.

SEATED LEG CURLS: work up to 3 sets of 10 reps. But on the last set, do a triple drop set, hitting 10 reps at each weight for a total of 40 reps on the last set. If you don't have a machine, use bands while sitting on a bench with the bands attached to a sturdy structure about 3–4 feet away. Perform the drop set by using progressively lighter bands. Rest 2–3 minutes between sets.

STANDING CALF RAISES: Warm up well, then do 4 sets of 25 reps.

SEATED CALF RAISES: 4 sets of 25 reps.

DONKEY CALF RAISES: You can perform these on a machine if your gym has one. Or, have a training partner (or two) sit on your back while you place your toes on a 4-by-4-inch block or something similar to increase your range of motion. With partners is how Arnold performed these back in the '70s. Do 4 sets of 25 reps.

WEEK THREE

DAY ONE: CHEST

INCLINE BARBELL PRESS: Use a low incline that is at an angle of approximately 15–20 degrees. Work up in 2–3 sets to a tough set of 6 reps and stay there for 4 sets of 6 reps. Rest 2–3 minutes between sets.

FLAT DUMBBELL PRESSES: Work up in 2–3 sets to a fairly tough set of 10 reps and stay there for 5 sets of 10 reps. Rest 2–3 minutes between sets.

PUSH-UPS WITH FEET ELEVATED AND WIDE HAND PLACEMENT: Put your feet up on a bench and keep your back and legs straight. Place your hands out wide and your elbows out to focus on your chest. Do three sets with just body weight until failure. Rest 2–3 minutes between sets.

DAY TWO: BACK

KROC ROWS: Do 2–3 warm up sets, then 1 × 20; go as heavy as possible on these (use straps) and try to beat your PR.

CHINS: Perform a total of 6 sets with body weight to failure. Vary the hand placement on each set. Start with a wide overhand grip; then use a medium, neutral grip; and finish with a close grip, using a V bar. Then start over with the wide grip so that you use each hand placement twice. If you can't get at least 10 reps per set, use a chin-assistance machine or bands to help you get the desired number of reps. Try to take the biceps out of the movement as much as possible and focus on using your lats throughout the movement. Rest 2–3 minutes between sets.

SEATED CABLE ROWS WITH A WIDE GRIP: Use a wide, straight bar as you would for wide-grip lat pull-downs and place your grip as far out as you can before the bar curves. Work up to a heavy set of 8 reps, and then stay there for 4 sets. Rest 2–3 minutes between sets.

BARBELL SHRUGS: Use straps and the heaviest weight possible (without using the rest of your body) and then just focus on moving your shoulders up and down (after warming up) for 3 sets of 20 reps. Rest 2–3 minutes between sets.

HYPEREXTENSIONS: Just use your body weight and go to complete failure, then rest 30 seconds and go to failure again. Rest 30 seconds and do one more set to failure. Push yourself on these, and then you're done for the day.

DAY THREE: SHOULDERS

SEATED DUMBBELL POWER CLEANS: After 1–2 warm-ups perform 3 sets of 20 reps. Do these by shrugging your shoulders up first. While holding them up, perform a clean-type movement to get the dumbbells above your shoulders, but don't attempt to dip under the weight. Instead, use your side and rear delts and traps to move the weight. Don't pause the weight in the top or bottom; just keep it moving up and down in a pumping motion. Rest 2–3 minutes between sets.

SEATED BENT-LATERAL RAISES: Perform 3 sets of 20 reps. Focus on using the rear delts and try to engage the traps as little as possible. Rest 2–3 minutes between sets.

SEATED DUMBBELL PRESSES: Work up slowly in sets of 6 reps until you reach your max set of 6. At least 4 of these should feel like work sets. Rest 2–3 minutes between sets.

DUMBBELL SHRUGS: Do 2–3 warm-up sets and then perform 4 sets of 25 reps with heavy dumbbells. Use straps here so that your grip isn't the limiting factor and just shrug the weight straight up and down with the greatest range of motion possible.

DAY FOUR: ARMS

DUMBBELL CURLS WITH PALMS UP: Do these curls one arm at a time. Warm up and then grab a weight that you have to work to get 10 reps with; perform all of your work sets with that.

> SUPERSETTED WITH:
>
> **DUMBBELL HAMMER CURLS:** Go immediately from dumbbell curls to these. Keep your elbows at your sides and, again, do all the reps with one arm before moving to the next.

Do 4 supersets of this combo, resting 2 minutes between supersets.

ROPE PUSHDOWNS: Keep your elbows at your sides and perform sets of 15 reps, pushing the rope apart at the bottom of the movement.

> SUPERSETTED WITH:
>
> **OVERHEAD ROPE EXTENSIONS:** Lighten the weight a bit, turn away from the machine, and do extensions out over your head. Do 15 reps of these as well.

Do 4 supersets of this combo, resting 2 minutes between supersets.

SEATED BARBELL CURLS: Do these with strict form and using a straight bar for sets of 15 reps.

> SUPERSETTED WITH:
>
> **STANDING BARBELL CURLS:** After completing 15 reps seated, stand up and do 10 more reps without a break. It is okay to use a little body English, but make sure the biceps are doing the work here.

Do 4 supersets of this combo, resting 2 minutes between supersets.

SKULL CRUSHERS WITH CHAINS: Load the EZ bar only with chains and set it up so that the chains are almost totally piled on the floor at the bottom of the movement but almost completely off the floor at lockout. Perform sets of 15 reps here.

CLOSE-GRIP BENCH WITH CHAINS: After your fifteenth rep on skulls, move the EZ bar to your chest and go directly into full-range, close-grip bench. Do 15 reps of these as well.

Do 4 supersets of this combo, resting 2 minutes between supersets, and you're done for the day. Your arms should be so swollen that they feel as if the skin is going to split.

DAY FIVE: LEGS

SQUATS WITH SAFETY-SQUAT BAR: (If you don't have one, just do traditional back squats.) Warm up and then work up to approximately 60–65% of your max. Next do 10 sets of 5 reps with only 45 seconds' rest between sets. It will seem easy at first and then get more difficult as the sets progress; by the end, you will barely be able to complete the reps on the last set.

LEG PRESS: Work up to a fairly difficult set of 10 reps in 2–3 sets. Stay there and do 5 sets of 10 reps with only 45 seconds' rest between sets. Don't lockout on these; just pump them up and down.

LEG EXTENSIONS: After warming up for a set or two, pick a weight that you have to work hard to get 30 reps with. Do 30 reps, then rest 30 seconds. Do 20 reps, then rest another 30 seconds. Do 10 more reps. Just do one set like this.

BARBELL STIFF-LEGGED DEADS: Keep your chest up and lower back arched and concentrate on using your hams to move the weight. Keep a slight bend in your knees throughout the movement. Do not rest the weight on the floor during the set; keep tension on the muscles at all times. Use 25-pound plates or stand on a platform to increase the range of motion. Work up to a hard set of 10 reps and then stay there for 4 sets of 10 reps. Rest 2–3 minutes between sets.

LYING LEG CURLS: work up to 3 sets of 10 reps. But on the last set, do a triple drop set, hitting 10 reps at each weight for a total of 40 reps

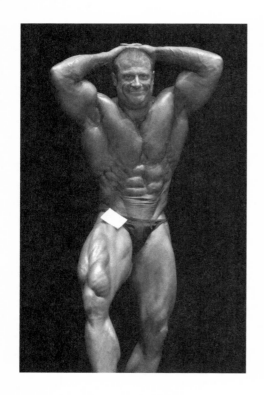

on the last set. If you don't have a machine, use bands while sitting on a bench with the bands attached to a sturdy structure about 3–4 feet away. Perform the drop set by using progressively lighter bands. Rest 2–3 minutes between sets.

CALF TRISET: After warming up a bit, start with calf raises on the leg-press machine and use a weight that allows 20 reps. Get off the leg press and immediately start doing standing calf raises off an elevated platform with just your body weight for 25 reps. Then go immediately to the seated calf machine and do another 20 reps. Repeat this three times, and you're done for the day. Rest 2–3 minutes between sets.

WEEK FOUR

DAY ONE: CHEST

REVERSE-BAND BENCH PRESS: Use medium to heavy bands that are hung from the top of a power rack. Warm up and work up to a max set of 5 reps. Work hard and try to set a new PR here. This should take 3–5 work sets, not counting warm-up sets. Rest 2–3 minutes between sets.

INCLINE DUMBBELL PRESSES: Use a low incline that is at an angle of approximately 15–25 degrees. In 2–3 sets, work up to a fairly tough set of 15 reps and stay there for 4 sets of 15 reps. Rest 2–3 minutes between sets.

LADDER PUSH-UPS: You can put a bar inside a power cage for these, setting pins at three different heights. Or, use a Smith machine if you have access to one. The first setting should be as low to the ground as possible. Pump out as many reps as you can, but stop 2–4 reps short of complete failure. Next move the bar up six to ten inches and pump out as many as possible, this time going to failure. Then move the bar up six to ten inches more and again go until failure. Your chest should be totally engorged with blood at this point. If you can do more than 25 reps on the first set, add resistance by having your training partners drape chains across your back in an X. Perform 3 sets, resting 2–3 minutes between them.

DAY TWO: BACK

ONE-ARM BARBELL ROWS: If you have a Meadows row handle, use it for these. If not, just grasp the barbell at the very end near the inside collar. Place the other end of the barbell in a landmine apparatus or shove it into a corner. Load just the one end of the barbell and use 25-pound or 10-pound plates on these to allow for a full range of motion. Work up to a hard set of 8 reps, then stay there for 4 sets. Rest 2–3 minutes between sets.

WIDE-OVERHAND-GRIP LAT PULL-DOWNS: Try to take the biceps out of the movement as much as possible and focus on using your lats throughout the movement. Work up to a hard set of 15 reps, then stay there for 4 sets. Rest 2–3 minutes between sets.

CHEST-SUPPORTED ROWS: Work up to a heavy set of 12 reps and then stay there for 4 sets. On the last set, perform a triple drop (48 reps total in the set) by stripping weight and doing 12 reps on each drop. Rest 2–3 minutes between sets.

DUMBBELL SHRUGS: Use straps and hold each rep at the top for 2 seconds with the traps fully contracted. Perform 3 sets of 10 reps. Rest 2–3 minutes between sets.

WEIGHTED HYPEREXTENSIONS: This week, add weight by holding a plate to your chest, placing chains around your neck, or, if you're really strong on these, by placing a barbell across your shoulders as you would in a high-bar squat position. Work up to a weight that's difficult for 10 reps and stay there for 3 sets of 10 reps. Rest 2–3 minutes between sets.

DAY THREE: SHOULDERS

SEATED CHAIN LATERAL RAISES: Clip D handles to chains and, after doing 1–2 warm-ups, perform 3 sets of 20 reps with a smooth and controlled tempo. On the last rep, hold the weight at lockout for as long as possible. Concentrate on using your medial delts to move the weight and avoid shrugging your shoulders up or back to keep the traps out of the movement as much as possible. Rest 2–3 minutes between sets.

BAND PULL-APARTS: Perform 4 sets of 25 reps. Focus on using the rear delts and try to engage the traps as little as possible. Rest 2–3 minutes between sets.

STANDING MILITARY PRESSES: Work up slowly in sets of 10 reps until you reach your max set of 10. At least 4 of these should feel like work sets. Rest 2–3 minutes between sets.

BARBELL SHRUGS: Perform 2–3 feeder sets and then do 5 sets of 10 reps, as heavy as possible. Just shrug the weight straight up and down since there is no reason to roll your shoulders or move them in a horizontal plane during the movement.

DAY FOUR: ARMS

BARBELL CURLS: Work up to a weight that's difficult for 20 reps. Stay there for 5 sets of 20 reps. Rest 2 minutes between sets.

V-BAR PUSHDOWNS: Work up to a weight that's difficult for 20 reps. Stay there for 5 sets of 20 reps. Rest 2 minutes between sets.

EZ-BAR PREACHER REVERSE CURLS: Start this superset with your palms facing down in a reverse-curl fashion. Perform 10 reps per set.

SUPERSETTED WITH:

EZ-BAR PREACHER CURLS: Reverse your grip so that your palms face up and keep going. Perform 10 reps per set.

Do 4 supersets of this combo, resting 2 minutes between them.

SKULL CRUSHERS WITH CHAINS: Load the EZ bar only with chains and set it up so that the chains are almost totally piled on the floor at the bottom of the movement but almost completely off the floor at lockout. Perform sets of 15 reps here.

> SUPERSETTED WITH:
>
> **CLOSE-GRIP BENCH WITH CHAINS:** After your fifteenth rep on skulls, move the EZ bar to your chest and go directly into full-range close-grip bench. Do 15 reps of these as well.

Do 4 supersets of this combo, resting 2 minutes between supersets. Your arms should be so swollen that they feel as if the skin is going to split.

DUMBBELL INCLINE CURLS: Perform 10 reps per set here, curling both dumbbells up at the same time with a smooth, controlled tempo.

> SUPERSETTED WITH:
>
> **DUMBBELL HAMMER CURLS:** Go immediately from dumbbell incline curls to these; just stand up and continue the set. Keep your elbows at your sides and curl both dumbbells at the same time, focusing on pumping up and down on the bottom half of the movement for 15 reps per set.

Do 4 supersets of this combo, resting 2 minutes between them.

REVERSE-GRIP PUSHDOWNS: Bend forward at the waist and bring the bar up above your head at the top of the rep. Only extend three quarters of the way at the bottom of the rep to work the stretch portion of the movement. Perform 15 reps per set of these.

> SUPERSETTED WITH:
>
> **CLOSE-GRIP PUSH-UPS:** Grab small hex dumbbells and use these as push-up stands. Place them about 8–12 inches apart and allow your palms to face each other. Keep your elbows tucked and focus on using your triceps throughout the movement. Perform each set to failure.

Do 4 supersets of this combo, resting 2 minutes between them.

DAY FIVE: LEGS

REVERSE-BAND SQUATS: Use medium or heavy bands suspended from the top of the squat rack for these. Warm up and then work up to a max set of 8 reps. And by "max," I mean that I want you to get the heaviest set of 8 reps that you can. This should take 3–5 work sets, not counting warm-up sets. Rest 2–4 minutes between sets.

LEG PRESS: Work up to a fairly difficult set of 20 reps—not an absolute max, but something you have to work for. Stay at that weight and do 5 sets of 20 reps. On your last set, you're really going to work hard and perform a long drop set. After the twentieth rep, have your training partner strip a plate off each side. Then, do 10 reps. Keep stripping one plate per side per set and doing 10 reps per set until the machine is empty. Rest 3–4 minutes between sets.

BULGARIAN SPLIT SQUATS: Put one foot up on a bench behind you with the other foot out front. Squat down on your front leg so that you're in a lunge-type position in the bottom and then push back up with your front leg. Perform 3 sets of 12 reps with each leg. Rest 2–3 minutes between sets.

DUMBBELL STIFF-LEGGED DEADS: Keep your chest up and lower back arched and concentrate on using your hams to move the weight. Keep a slight bend in your knees throughout the movement. Do not rest the weight on the floor during the set; keep tension on the muscles at all times. Work up to a hard set of 15 reps and then stay there for 4 sets of 15 reps. Rest 2–3 minutes between sets.

SEATED LEG CURLS: 4 sets of 25 reps. If you don't have a machine, use bands while sitting on a bench with the bands attached to a sturdy structure about 3–4 feet away. Hook the bands behind your ankles. Rest 2–3 minutes between sets.

STANDING CALF RAISES: Warm up well, then do 4 sets of 25 reps.

SEATED CALF RAISES: Perform 4 sets of 25 reps.

DONKEY CALF RAISES: You can perform these on a machine if your gym has one. Or, have a training partner (or two) sit on your back while placing your toes on a four-by-four-inch block or something similar to increase your range of motion. With partners is how Arnold performed these back in the '70s. Do 4 sets of 25 reps.

WEEK FIVE

DAY ONE: CHEST

INCLINE BARBELL PRESS: Use a low incline that is at an angle of approximately 15–20 degrees. Work up in 2–3 sets to a tough set of 8 reps and stay there for 4 sets of 8 reps. Rest 2–3 minutes between sets.

DUMBBELL TWIST PRESSES: Perform these by starting just as you would for a traditional dumbbell bench press. As you press the weight up, however, twist your wrists so that, at the top of the movement, your palms are supinated like a reverse-grip bench press. Then touch the ends of the dumbbells together. Start light and work up in small increments for sets of 10 reps until you can no longer fully rotate the dumbbells at the top. This is much harder than a regular dumbbell bench press. At least 4 of these sets should be work sets. Rest 2–3 minutes between sets.

WEIGHTED DIPS: Lean forward on these and focus on using your chest, not your triceps, to move the weight. Avoid fully locking out to keep the tension on the chest. Work up to a set of 10 reps with as much weight as possible. Stay there for 3 sets of 10 reps; on the last set, do a triple drop set. That is, after doing your 10 reps, drop enough weight to allow you to do 10 more reps with effort; then drop all the weight and do 10 more reps with just your body weight. Rest 2–3 minutes between sets.

DAY TWO: BACK

ONE-ARM BARBELL ROWS: If you have a Meadows row handle, use it for these. If not, just grasp the barbell at the very end near the inside collar. Place the other end of the barbell in a landmine apparatus or shove it into a corner. Load just the one end of the barbell and use 25-pound or 10-pound plates on these to allow for a full range of motion. Work up to a hard set of 10 reps, then stay there for 4 sets. Rest 2–3 minutes between sets.

CHINS: Perform 3 sets of 20 reps. Vary the hand placement on each set. Start with a wide overhand grip; then use a medium, neutral grip; and finish with a close grip, using a V bar. If you can't get 20 reps per set, use a chin-assistance machine or bands to help you get the desired number of reps. Try to take the biceps out of the movement as much as possible and focus on using your lats throughout the movement. Rest 2–3 minutes between sets.

T-BAR ROWS: Use a V handle with a barbell in a landmine-type device or with the end of the barbell shoved in a corner. Work up a 45 pound plate (or 25-pound plate at a time depending on your strength level) at 10 reps per set until you can no longer get 10 reps. At least 4 of these should be work sets. Rest 2–3 minutes between sets.

BARBELL SHRUGS: Use straps and the heaviest weight possible (without using the rest of your body). Focus on moving your shoulders up and down (after warming up) for 3 sets of 20 reps. Rest 2–3 minutes between sets.

BANDED HYPEREXTENSIONS: Use a shortened light band and put it over your head around your neck. Perform 30 sets of 20 reps but make the last a drop set by doing your 20 reps and then dropping the band and going until failure. Rest 2–3 minutes between sets.

DAY THREE: SHOULDERS

SHOULDER COMPLEX: This is performed seated with dumbbells and consists of one big triset of three exercises performed consecutively and without rest in between. Start with front raises. Next do lateral raises. Finish with seated bent laterals. Do 20 reps of each exercise for a total of 60 reps per set. Perform 3 sets, resting 2–3 minutes between sets.

BAND PULL-APARTS: Perform 4 sets of 25 reps. Focus on using the rear delts and try to engage the traps as little as possible. Rest 2–3 minutes between sets.

SEATED DUMBBELL PRESSES: Work up slowly in sets of 8 reps until you reach your max set of 8. At least 4 of these should feel like work sets. Rest 2–3 minutes between sets.

DUMBBELL SHRUGS: Do 2–3 warm-up sets and then perform 4 sets of 25 reps with heavy dumbbells. Use straps here so that your grip isn't the limiting factor and just shrug the weight straight up and down with the greatest range of motion possible.

DAY FOUR: ARMS

DOWN-THE-RACK BARBELL CURLS: Warm up, then start with a weight that you can get 10 reps with but still have 2–3 reps in the tank. As soon as you get to 10, either strip some weight (loading all 10-pound or 5-pound plates on a barbell works well) or grab a barbell that is approximately 10–20% lighter and do another 10 reps. Then do three more drops, performing 10 reps at each drop for a total of 4 drops, which equals 5 sets for a total of 50 reps. Your arms should be totally filled with blood from just one long drop set of this.

STRAIGHT-BAR-PUSHDOWN DROP SET: Using the same method as above, warm up and then complete a set of 10 reps with a weight that, at most, would allow you to do 12–13 reps. Then immediately move the pin up a couple holes and do 10 more reps. Keep doing this for a total of 5 drop sets, equaling 50 reps.

CABLE CURLS: Use a curl-bar attachment on the low pulley. Use a weight that you can get about 20 reps with, but only do 15 reps. Do this for 5 sets. The kicker is that you'll only be resting for 45 seconds between sets. Your arms will swell huge from the high volume and short rest periods.

LYING EXTENSIONS WITH CHAINS: Lie flat on your back and perform a skull-crusher-type movement with chains. These can be clipped to D handles or the grenade handles from Elitefts if you have them. Perform 5 sets of 10 reps with only 45 seconds' rest between sets.

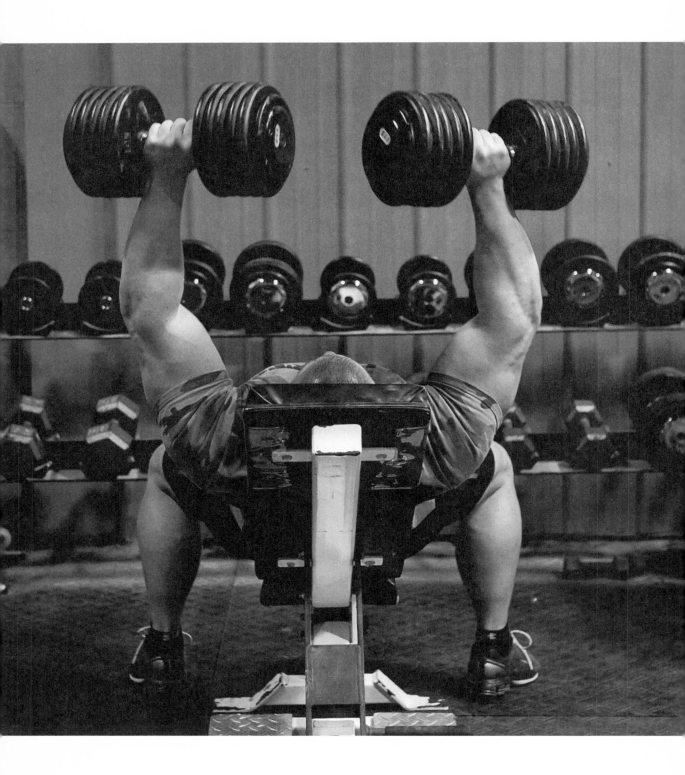

REVERSE CURLS WITH EZ-CURL BAR: Use a weight that you can get about 20 reps with, but only do 15 reps. Do this for 5 sets. Again, the kicker is that you'll only be resting for 45 seconds between sets. Your biceps and forearms will swell huge from the high volume and short rest periods.

OVERHEAD CABLE EXTENSIONS: Use a rope handle attached to the high pulley. Face away from the machine and bend over at the waist. Extend the rope from behind your head straight out in front of you to arm's length. Perform 5 sets of 10 reps with only 45 seconds' rest between sets.

DAY FIVE: LEGS

SQUATS WITH SAFETY-SQUAT BAR: (If you don't have one, just do traditional back squats.) Warm up and then work up to approximately 60–65% of your max, just as you did a couple of weeks ago. This time, use at least 10 pounds more than you used in week three. Now do 10 sets of 5 reps with only 45 seconds' rest between sets.

LEG PRESS: Do 2–3 sets, working up to a weight that requires you to really work to get 20 reps. You are only going to do one all-out work set here, but the trick to this is to find a way to get 40 reps with a weight that would be difficult to get 20 with. Pause at lockout, push with your hands on your knees—do whatever you have to do to get all 40 reps in one set without racking the weight. Really push yourself here and resist the temptation to wimp out and take a weight you know you can do.

CHAIN LUNGES: Throw the appropriate amount of chains around your neck and take 30 steps (15 reps with each leg), touching your knee to the ground on each step. Do this for 3 sets of 30 steps. Rest 2–3 minutes between sets.

BARBELL STIFF-LEGGED DEADS: Keep your chest up and lower back arched and concentrate on using your hams to move the weight. Keep a slight bend in your knees throughout the movement. Do not rest the weight on the floor during the set; keep tension on the muscles at all times. Use 25-pound plates or stand on a platform to increase the range of motion. Work up to a hard set of 10 reps and then stay there for 4 sets of 10 reps. Rest 2–3 minutes between sets.

LYING LEG CURLS: work up to 4 sets of 25 reps. If you don't have a machine, use bands while sitting on a bench with the bands attached to a sturdy structure about 3–4 feet away. Rest 2–3 minutes between sets.

CALF TRISET: After warming up a bit, start with calf raises on the leg-press machine and use a weight that allows 20 reps. Get off the leg press and immediately start doing standing calf raises off an elevated platform with just your body weight for twenty-five reps. Then go immediately to the seated calf machine and do another 20 reps. Repeat this three times, and you're done for the day. Rest 2–3 minutes between sets.

WEEK SIX

DAY TWO: CHEST

INCLINE DUMBBELL PRESSES: Use a low incline that is at an angle of approximately 15–25 degrees. Work up in 2–3 sets to a fairly tough set of 10 reps and stay there for 4 sets of 10 reps. Rest 2–3 minutes between sets.

STANDARD BENCH PRESS: After a warm-up set or two, take a weight at or close to your 5-rep max. Then perform 5 sets of 5 reps, but decrease the weight on the bar by 10 pounds each set. If your 5-rep max was 400×5, your session would look like this: 400×5, 390×5, 380×5, 370×5, 360×5. Rest 2–3 minutes between sets.

PUSH-UPS WITH FEET ELEVATED AND WIDE HAND PLACEMENT: Put your feet up on a bench and keep your back and legs straight. Place your hands out wide and your elbows out to focus on your chest. Do three sets with just body weight until failure. Rest 2–3 minutes between sets.

DAY TWO: BACK

KROC ROWS: Do 2–3 warm-up sets and then 1×20. Go as heavy as possible on these (use straps) and try to beat your PR.

CHINS: Perform a total of 6 sets with body weight to failure. Vary the hand placement on each set. Start with a wide overhand grip; then use a medium, neutral grip; and finish with a close grip, using a V bar. Then start over with the wide grip so that you use each hand placement twice. If you can't get at least 10 reps per set, use a chin-assistance machine or bands to help you get the desired number of reps. Try to take the biceps out of the movement as much as possible and focus on using your lats throughout the movement. Rest 2–3 minutes between sets.

CHEST-SUPPORTED ROWS: Work up to a heavy set of 12 reps and then stay there for 4 sets. On the last set, perform a triple drop (48 reps total in the set) by stripping weight and doing 12 reps on each drop. Rest 2–3 minutes between sets.

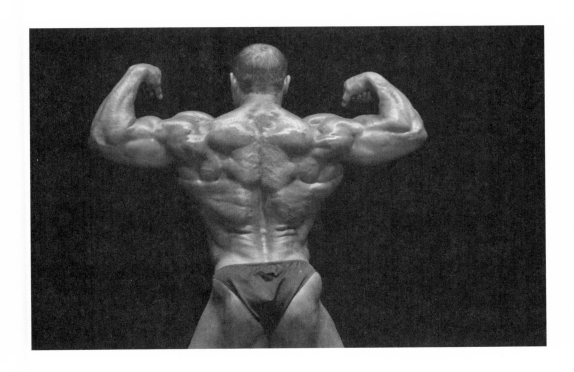

DUMBBELL SHRUGS: Use straps and hold each rep at the top for 2 seconds with the traps fully contracted. Perform 3 sets of 10 reps. Rest 2–3 minutes between sets.

HYPEREXTENSIONS: Use your body weight and go to complete failure. Then rest 30 seconds and go to failure again. Rest 30 seconds and do one more set to failure. Push yourself on these, and then you're done for the day.

DAY THREE: SHOULDERS

SEATED DUMBBELL POWER CLEANS: After 1–2 warm-ups, perform 3 sets of 20 reps. Do these sitting at the end of a bench. Start by shrugging your shoulders up first. While holding them up, perform a clean-type movement to get the dumbbells above your shoulders, but don't attempt to dip under the weight. Instead, use your side and rear delts and traps to move the weight. Don't pause the weight in the top or bottom; just keep it moving up and down in a pumping motion. Rest 2–3 minutes between sets.

DUMBBELL BENT LATERALS: Sit on the end of a flat bench and bend forward far enough to allow the dumbbells to touch under your legs at the bottom of the movement. Perform 3 sets of 20 reps. Again, focus on using the rear delts and try to engage the traps as little as possible. Rest 2–3 minutes between sets.

STANDING MILITARY PRESSES: Work up slowly in sets of 12 reps until you reach your max set of 12. At least 4 of these should feel like work sets. Rest 2–3 minutes between sets.

BARBELL SHRUGS: Perform 2–3 feeder sets and then do 5 sets of 10 reps, as heavy as possible. Just shrug the weight straight up and down since there is no reason to roll your shoulders or move them in a horizontal plane during the movement.

DAY FOUR: ARMS

Today you will perform trisets for biceps and triceps. This is a series of three exercises performed consecutively with no rest in between. You then rest 2–3 minutes before doing the next triset. You will perform 3 tri-sets for each series for a total of 9 sets for each body part.

TRISET FOR BICEPS: Do EZ-bar curls × 20 reps; then do EZ–bar reverse curls × 10 reps; next perform dumbbell hammer curls (both arms at same time) × 10 reps.

TRISET FOR TRICEPS: First perform dumbbell incline extensions × 15 reps; then do pushdowns × 15 reps; and finish with bench dips until failure.

After trisets are complete, finish today's training with one standard exercise for biceps and one for triceps.

CABLE CURLS: Perform 5 sets of 10 reps with only 60 seconds' rest in between sets.

SKULL CRUSHERS WITH CHAINS: Load the EZ bar only with chains and set it up so that the chains are almost totally piled on the floor at the bottom of the movement but almost completely off the floor at lockout. Perform 5 sets of 10 reps with only 60 seconds' rest in between sets.

DAY FIVE: LEGS

SQUATS: Just do regular old back squats today. Warm up and work up slowly to a weight that is your true 5-rep max. Work hard and go for a PR here. This should take 3–5 working sets. Rest 2–3 minutes between sets.

LEG PRESS: This is another brutal up-and-down set. First work up to a weight that is about 60% of your 10-rep max, and then you will do one all-out up-and-down set. This is how it works: perform 5 reps with the 60% and then hold the weight at lockout (the weight is never racked until all the sets are done) and have your training partners add a plate to each side and do another 5 reps; then hold it at lockout as they add another plate to each side. Keep doing 5 reps at each weight and going up until you can barely get 5 reps (this should take at least 4–5 sets). Even though your legs will be on fire, you're only halfway done. Next have your partners start stripping weights a plate at a time and do 5 reps at each weight until you get back down to where you started. Your legs should be burning like never before. You should be able to perform around 10 sets total with about 50 total reps.

BULGARIAN SPLIT SQUATS WITH CHAINS: Put one foot up on a bench behind you with the other foot out front. Squat down on your front leg so that you're in a lunge-type position in the bottom and then push back up with your front leg. Add resistance by placing chains around your neck. Perform 4 sets of 8 reps with each leg. Rest 2–3 minutes between sets.

DUMBBELL STIFF-LEGGED DEADS: Keep your chest up and lower back arched and concentrate on using your hams to move the weight. Keep a slight bend in your knees throughout the movement. Do not rest the weight on the floor during the set; keep tension on the muscles at all times. Work up to a hard set of 20 reps and then stay there for 4 sets of 20 reps. Rest 2–3 minutes between sets.

SEATED LEG CURLS: work up to 3 sets of 10 reps. But on the last set, do a triple drop set, hitting 10 reps at each weight for a total of 40 reps on the last set. If you don't have a machine, use bands while sitting on a bench with the bands attached to a sturdy structure about 3–4 feet away. Perform the drop set by using progressively lighter bands. Rest 2–3 minutes between sets.

STANDING CALF RAISES: Warm up well, then do 4 sets of 25 reps.

SEATED CALF RAISES: Perform 4 sets of 25 reps.

DONKEY CALF RAISES: You can perform these on a machine if your gym has one. Or, have a training partner (or two) sit on your back while you place your toes on a four-by-four-inch block or something similar to increase your range of motion. With partners is how Arnold performed these back in the '70s. Again, do 4 sets of 25 reps.

WEEK SEVEN

DAY ONE: CHEST

CHAIN BENCH PRESS: Use approximately 100 pounds in chains and then add plates at each set to increase the weight. Warm up and work up to a max set of 5 reps. Work hard and try to set a new PR here. This should take 3-5 work sets, not counting warm-up sets. Rest 2–4 minutes between sets.

INCLINE BARBELL PRESSES: Use a low incline that is at an angle of approximately 15–25 degrees. Work up in 2–3 sets to a fairly tough set of 5 reps and stay there for 5 sets of 5 reps. Rest 2–3 minutes between sets.

LADDER PUSH-UPS: You can put a bar inside a power cage for these, setting pins at three different heights. Or, use a Smith machine if you have access to one. The first setting should be as low to the ground as possible. Pump out as many reps as you can, stopping 2–4 reps short of complete failure. Now move the bar up six to ten inches and pump out as many as possible, this time going to failure. Then move the bar up another six to ten inches and go again until failure. Your chest should be totally engorged with blood at this point. If you can do more than 25 reps on the first set, add resistance by having your training partners drape chains across your back in an X. Perform 3 sets, resting 2–3 minutes between sets.

DAY TWO: BACK

ONE-ARM BARBELL ROWS: If you have a Meadows row handle, use it for these. If not, just grasp the barbell at the very end near the inside collar. Place the other end of the barbell in a landmine apparatus or shove it into a corner. Load just the one end of the barbell and use 25- pound or 10-pound plates on these to allow for a full range of motion. Work up to a max set of 10 reps. Work hard and set a PR here. At least 3–4 sets should be work sets. Rest 2–3 minutes between sets.

WIDE-OVERHAND-GRIP LAT PULL-DOWNS: Try to take the biceps out of the movement as much as possible and focus on using your lats throughout the movement. After two feeder sets, pick a weight that will require you to work hard to get 25 reps, then stay there for 4 sets. Rest 2–3 minutes between sets.

T-BAR ROWS: Use a V bar with a barbell in a landmine-type device or with the end of the barbell shoved in a corner. Work up a 45 pound plate (or 25-pound plate at a time depending on your strength level) at 10 reps per set until you can no longer get 10 reps. At least 4 of these should be work sets. Rest 2–3 minutes between sets.

BARBELL SHRUGS: Use a double overhand grip and focus on moving your shoulders up and down (after warming up), using as much weight as possible for 3 sets of 20 reps.

HYPEREXTENSIONS: Using your body weight, do one all-out balls-to-the-wall set to failure. Push yourself on these, get a PR, and then you're done for the day.

DAY THREE: SHOULDERS

LEANING LATERAL RAISES: Grab onto a sturdy structure with one hand and hold the dumbbell in the other. Keeping your feet together and close to the structure, lean away from it until your arm is straight. This will make the movement very strict and hit the medial delt hard. After 1–2 warm-ups, perform 3 sets of 15 reps with a smooth and controlled tempo. Rest 2–3 minutes between sets.

BAND PULL-APARTS: Perform 4 sets of 25 reps. Focus on using the rear delts and try to engage the traps as little as possible. Rest 1–2 minutes between sets.

SEATED DUMBBELL PRESSES: Work up slowly in sets of 10 reps until you reach your max set of 10. At least 4 of these should feel like work sets. Rest 2–3 minutes between sets.

DUMBBELL SHRUGS: Do 2–3 warm-up sets and then perform 4 sets of 25 reps with heavy dumbbells. Use straps here so that your grip isn't the limiting factor and just shrug the weight straight up and down with the greatest range of motion possible.

DAY FOUR: ARMS

This may be the most challenging arm day yet. This is what I call my 1,000-rep arm workout. It consists of ten exercises, all 5 sets of 20 reps. It is okay to lighten the weights after the first few exercises to ensure you do all the reps. The priority here is completing every rep inside the prescribed rest periods, not the amount of weight used. Enjoy!!!

EZ-BAR CURLS: After a few warm-up sets, perform 5 sets of 20 reps with 2–3 minutes of rest between sets.

STRAIGHT BAR PUSHDOWNS: After a few warm-up sets, perform 5 sets of 20 reps with 2–3 minutes of rest between sets. Keep your elbows glued to your sides and don't pause the reps; just pump them up and down.

CABLE CURLS: Use an EZ-curl-shaped handle and attach it to the lower cable. Perform 5 sets of 20 reps with 2–3 minutes of rest between sets.

OVERHEAD CABLE EXTENSIONS: Use a rope handle attached to the high pulley. Face away from the machine and bend over at the waist, extending the rope from behind your head straight out in front of you to arm's length. Perform 5 sets of 20 reps with 2–3 minutes of rest between sets.

DUMBBELL HAMMER CURLS: Keep your elbows at your sides and, again, do all the reps with both arms at the same time. Perform 5 sets of 20 reps with 2–3 minutes of rest between sets.

LYING EXTENSIONS WITH CHAINS: Lie flat on your back and perform a skull-crusher-type movement with chains. These can be with an EZ-curl bar or with the chains clipped to D handles or the grenade handles from Elitefts if you have them. Perform 5 sets of 20 reps with 2–3 minutes of rest between sets.

SEATED BARBELL CURLS: Use a straight barbell for these and perform them strictly, touching your thighs at the bottom of the movement but not resting the weight on them. Perform 5 sets of 20 reps with 2–3 minutes of rest between sets.

DUMBBELL KICKBACKS: Bend over at the waist and extend both arms at the same time. Keep your upper arms parallel to the floor and pause the reps briefly at the top with full extension while flexing the triceps. Perform 5 sets of 20 reps with only 1–2 minutes of rest between sets.

EZ-BAR REVERSE CURLS: Keep your form strict here and limit the amount of body swing, using lighter weights if necessary since your arms should be completely fried by this point. Perform 5 sets of 20 reps with 2–3 minutes of rest between sets.

BENCH DIPS: Body weight is all you should need by the time you get here. Set up two benches of the same height. Perform dips in between them, keeping your legs straight, your feet on one bench, and your hands on the bench just behind you. Perform 5 sets of 20 reps with only 1–2 minutes of rest between sets.

DAY FIVE: LEGS

REVERSE BAND SQUATS: Use medium or heavy bands suspended from the top of the squat rack for these. Warm up and then work up to a max set of 6 reps. By "max," I mean that I want you to get the heaviest set of 6 reps that you can. This should take 3–5 work sets, not counting warm-up sets. Rest 2–4 minutes between sets.

LEG PRESS: Today you are going to do lots of reps. After 1–2 medium warm-up feeder sets, pick a weight that will require you to work hard to get 25 reps and stay here for 4 sets of 25 reps (100 reps total). Rest 2–4 minutes between sets.

LEG EXTENSIONS: Again, do 1–2 feeder sets and then pick a weight that challenges you for 3 sets of 30 reps. Rest 2–3 minutes between sets.

BARBELL STIFF-LEGGED DEADS: Use 25-pound plates for these or stand on a four-inch platform to increase the range of motion. Keep

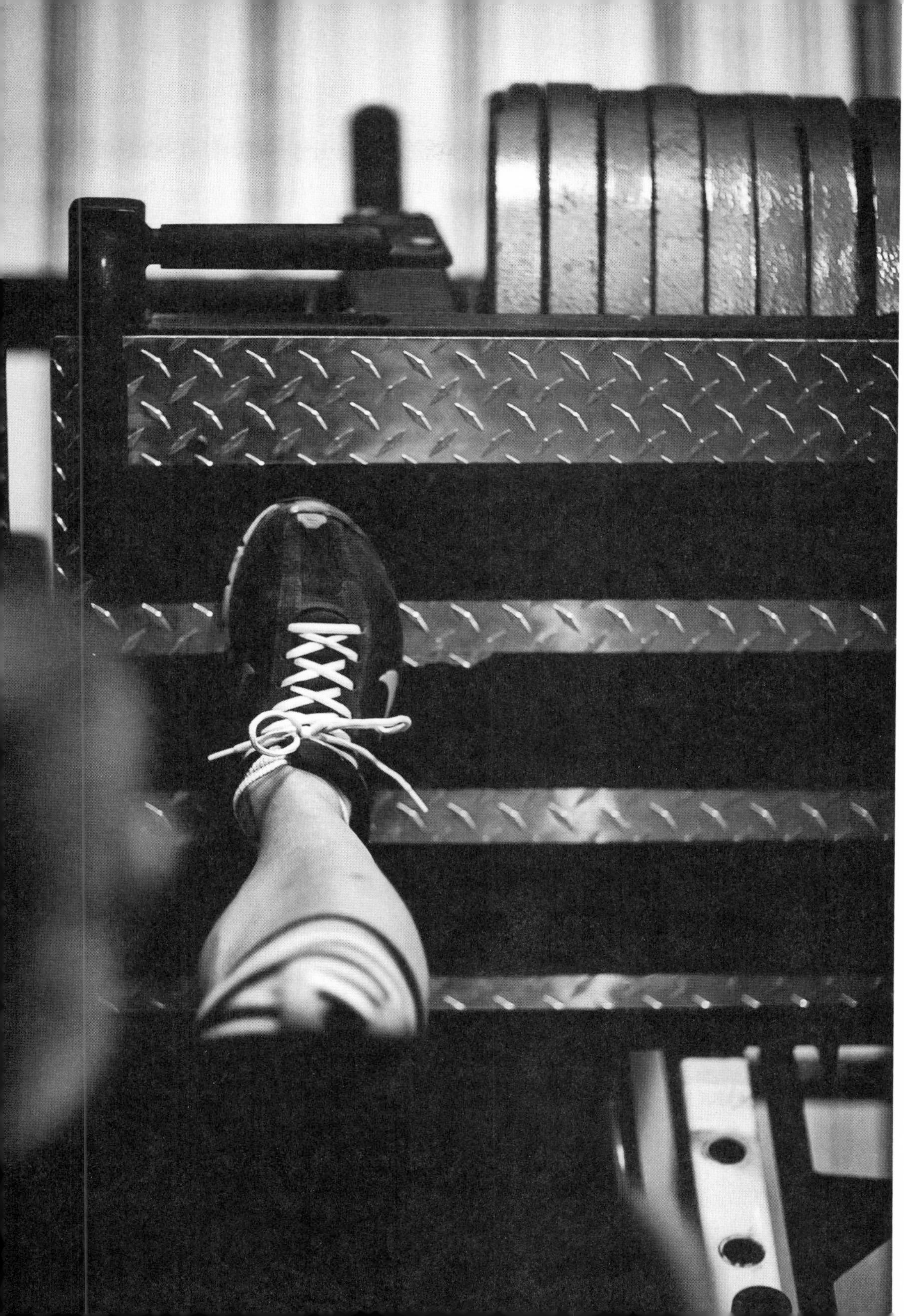

your chest up and lower back arched and concentrate on using your hams to move the weight. Keep a slight bend in your knees throughout the movement. Do not rest the weight on the floor during the set; keep tension on the muscles at all times. Work up to a hard set of 8 reps and then stay there for 4 sets of 8 reps. Rest 2–3 minutes between sets.

LYING LEG CURLS: work up to 3 sets of 10 reps. But on the last set, do a triple drop set, hitting 10 reps at each weight for a total of 40 reps on the last set. Rest 2–3 minutes between sets.

CALF TRISET: After warming up a bit, start with calf raises on the leg-press machine, using a weight that allows 20 reps. Get off the leg press and immediately start doing standing calf raises off an elevated platform with just your body weight for 25 reps. Then go immediately to the seated calf machine and do another 20 reps. Repeat this three times, and you're done for the day. Rest 2–3 minutes between sets.

WEEK EIGHT

DAY ONE: CHEST

FLAT DUMBBELL PRESSES: Warm up and work up to a max set of 8 reps. Work hard and try to set a new PR here. This should take 3–5 work sets, not counting warm-up sets. Rest 2–3 minutes between sets.

INCLINE BARBELL PRESS: Today we will perform what I refer to as a reverse pyramid. Use a low incline that is at an angle of approximately 15–20 degrees. Work up in 2–3 sets to a tough set of 5 reps. Decrease the weight by 10% and do a set of 10 reps. Then decrease the weight by 10% and do a set of 15 reps. Then decrease the weight by 10% and do a set of 20 reps. Rest 2–3 minutes between sets.

WEIGHTED DIPS: Lean forward on these and focus on using your chest, not your triceps, to move the weight. Avoid fully locking out to keep the tension on the chest. Work up to a set of 10 reps with as much weight as possible. Stay there for 3 sets of 10 reps; on the last set, do a triple drop set. So do your 10 reps and then drop enough weight to allow you to do 10 more reps with effort. Then drop all the weight and do 10 more reps with just your body weight. Rest 2–3 minutes between sets.

DAY TWO: BACK

BARBELL ROWS: You can be a little loose with the form here and do these rows with some upper back movement to get the bar moving. Work up slowly to a max set of 10 reps. Work hard and try set a PR here. At least 3–4 sets should be work sets. Rest 2–3 minutes between sets.

CHINS: Perform a total of 6 sets with body weight to failure. Vary the hand placement on each set. Start with a wide overhand grip; then use a medium, neutral grip; and finish with a close grip using a V bar. Then start over with the wide grip so that you use each hand placement twice. If you can't get at least 10 reps per set, use a chin-assistance machine or bands to help you get the desired number of reps. Try to take the biceps out of the movement as much as possible and focus on using your lats throughout the movement. Rest 2–3 minutes between sets.

T-BAR ROWS: Use a V bar with a barbell in a landmine-type device or with the end of the barbell shoved in a corner. Work up a 45 pound plate (or 25-pound plate at a time depending on your strength level) at 10 reps per set until you can no longer get 10 reps. At least 4 of these should be work sets. Rest 2–3 minutes between sets.

DUMBBELL SHRUGS: Use straps and hold each rep at the top for 2 seconds with the traps fully contracted. Perform 3 sets of 10 reps. Rest 2–3 minutes between sets.

BANDED HYPEREXTENSIONS: Use a shortened light band and put it over your head and around your neck. Perform 3 sets of 20 reps. Make the last set a drop set by doing your 20 reps and then dropping the band and going until failure. Rest 2–3 minutes between sets.

DAY THREE: SHOULDERS

SEATED DUMBBELL POWER CLEANS: After 1–2 warm-ups, perform 3 sets of 20 reps. Do these by shrugging your shoulders up first. While holding them up, perform a clean-type movement to get the dumbbells above your shoulders, but don't attempt to dip under the weight. Instead, use your side and rear delts and traps to move the weight. Don't pause the weight at the top or bottom; just keep it moving up and down in a pumping motion. Rest 2–3 minutes between sets.

SEATED BENT-LATERAL RAISES: Perform 3 sets of 20 reps. Focus on using the rear delts and try to engage the traps as little as possible. Rest 2–3 minutes between sets.

STANDING MILITARY PRESSES: This is another reverse pyramid. Work up in 2–3 sets to a tough set of 5 reps. Decrease the weight by 10–15% and do a set of 10 reps. Then decrease the weight by 10–15% and do a set of 15 reps. Then decrease the weight by 10–15% and do a set of 20 reps. Rest 2–3 minutes between sets.

BARBELL SHRUGS: Perform 2–3 feeder sets and then do 5 sets of 10 reps, as heavy as possible. Just shrug the weight straight up and down since there is no reason to roll your shoulders or move them in a horizontal plane during the movement.

DAY FOUR: ARMS

DUMBBELL CURLS WITH PALMS UP: Curl these one arm at a time and keep your hand supinated (palm up) the entire time. Warm up, then grab a weight that you have to work to get 10 reps with and perform all of your work sets with that.

SUPERSETTED WITH:

DUMBBELL HAMMER CURLS: Go immediately from dumbbell curls to these. Keep your elbows at your sides and, again, do all the reps with one arm before moving to the next (10 reps with each arm).

Do 4 supersets of this combo, resting 2 minutes between supersets.

ROPE PUSHDOWNS: Keep your elbows at your sides and perform sets of 15 reps, pushing the rope apart at the bottom of the movement.

SUPERSETTED WITH:

OVERHEAD ROPE EXTENSIONS: Lighten the weight a bit, turn away from the machine, and do extensions out over your head. Do 15 reps of these as well.

Do 4 supersets of this combo, resting 2 minutes between supersets.

SEATED BARBELL CURLS: Do these with strict form and using a straight bar for sets of 15 reps.

SUPERSETTED WITH:

STANDING BARBELL CURLS: After completing 15 reps seated, stand up and do 10 more reps without a break. It is okay to use a little body English, but make sure the biceps are doing the work here.

Do 4 supersets of this combo resting 2 minutes between supersets.

SKULL CRUSHERS WITH CHAINS: Load the EZ bar only with chains and set it up so that the chains are almost totally piled on the floor at the bottom of the movement but almost completely off the floor at lockout. Perform sets of 15 reps.

SUPERSETTED WITH:

CLOSE-GRIP BENCH WITH CHAINS: After your fifteenth rep on skulls, just move the EZ bar to your chest and go directly into full-range, close-grip bench. Do 15 reps of these as well.

After doing 4 supersets of this combo—resting 2 minutes between supersets—you're done for the day. Your arms should be so swollen that they feel as if the skin is going to split.

DAY FIVE: LEGS

SQUATS WITH SAFETY-SQUAT BAR: (If you don't have one, just do traditional back squats.) Warm up and then work up to approximately 60–65% of your max, just as you did a couple of weeks ago. This time, use at least 10 pounds more than you used in week 5. Do 10 sets of 5 reps with only 45 seconds' rest between sets.

LEG PRESS: Perform what I call an up-and-down set. In case you don't remember exactly how to do it from before, here's a reminder. First work up to a weight that is about 60% of your 10-rep max and then do one all-out up-and-down set. This is how it works: perform 5 reps with the 60% and then hold the weight at lockout (the weight is never racked until all the sets are done) and have your training partners add a plate to each side and do another 5 reps; then hold it at lockout as they add another plate to each side. Keep doing 5 reps at each weight and going up until you can barely get 5 reps (this should take at least 4–5 sets). Even though your legs will be on fire, you're only halfway done. Next have your partners start stripping weights a plate at a time and do 5 reps at each weight until you get back down to where you started. Your legs should be burning like never before. You should be able to perform around 10 sets total with about 50 total reps.

BULGARIAN SPLIT SQUATS: Put one foot up on a bench behind you with the other foot out front. Squat down on your front leg so that you're in a lunge-type position in the bottom and then push back up with your front leg. If the squats are too easy with just body weight, add resistance by placing chains around your neck. After the first two movements, however, I seriously doubt they will be too easy. Perform 4 sets of 15 reps with each leg. Rest 2–3 minutes between sets.

DUMBBELL STIFF-LEGGED DEADS: Keep your chest up and lower back arched and concentrate on using your hams to move the weight. Keep a slight bend in your knees throughout the movement. Do not rest the weight on the floor during the set; keep tension on the muscles at all times. Work up to a hard set of 20 reps and then stay there for 4 sets of 20 reps. Rest 2–3 minutes between sets.

SEATED LEG CURLS: work up to 3 sets of 20 reps. If you don't have a machine, use bands while sitting on a bench with the bands attached to a sturdy structure about 3–4 feet away. Rest 2–3 minutes between sets.

STANDING CALF RAISES: Warm up well, then do 4 sets of 25 reps.

SEATED CALF RAISES: Do 4 sets of 25 reps.

DONKEY CALF RAISES: You can perform these on a machine if your gym has one. Or, have a training partner (or two) sit on your back while placing your toes on a four-by-four-inch block or something similar to increase your range of motion. With partners is how Arnold performed these back in the '70s. Again, do 4 sets of 25 reps.

WEEK NINE

DAY ONE: CHEST

CHAIN BENCH PRESS: Use approximately 100 pounds in chains and then add plates before each set to increase the weight. Warm up and work up to a max set of 8 reps. Work hard and try to set a new PR here. This should take 3–5 work sets, not counting warm-up sets. Rest 2–4 minutes between sets.

INCLINE BARBELL PRESSES: Use a low incline that is only at an angle of approximately 15–25 degrees. Work up in 2–3 sets to a fairly tough set of 10 reps and stay there for 5 sets of 10 reps. Rest 2–3 minutes between sets.

PUSH-UPS WITH FEET ELEVATED AND WIDE HAND PLACEMENT: Put your feet up on a bench and keep your back and legs straight. Place your hands out wide and your elbows out to focus on your chest. Do three sets with just body weight until failure. Rest 2–3 minutes between sets.

DAY TWO: BACK

KROC ROWS: Do 2–3 warm-up sets and then 1 x 20; go as heavy as possible on these (use straps) and try to beat your PR.

WIDE-NEUTRAL-GRIP LAT PULL-DOWNS: Use a ladder-bar-type attachment that allows you to take a wide neutral grip. Try to take the biceps out of the movement as much as possible and focus on using your lats throughout the movement. After two feeder sets, pick a weight that will require you to work hard to get 10 reps, then stay there for 4 sets of 10 reps. Rest 2–3 minutes between sets.

CHEST-SUPPORTED ROWS: Work up to a heavy set of 12 reps and then stay there for 4 sets. On the last set, perform a triple drop (48 reps total in the set) by stripping weight and doing 12 reps on each drop. Rest 2–3 minutes between sets.

BARBELL SHRUGS: Use a double overhand grip and hold each rep at the top for 3 seconds for 3 sets of 10 reps.

HYPEREXTENSIONS: Just use your body weight and go to complete failure, then stay on the bench. Rest 30 seconds and go to failure again. Rest 30 seconds and do one more set to failure. Push yourself on these, and then you're done for the day.

DAY THREE: SHOULDERS

SEATED CHAIN LATERAL RAISES: Clip D handles to chains and, after 1–2 warm-ups, perform 3 sets of 20 reps with a smooth and controlled tempo. On the last rep, hold the weight at lockout for as long as possible. Concentrate on using your medial delts to move the weight. Avoid shrugging your shoulders up or back to keep the traps out of the movement as much as possible. Rest 2–3 minutes between sets.

SEATED DUMBBELL POWER CLEANS: After 1–2 warm-ups, perform 3 sets of 20 reps. Do these by shrugging your shoulders up first. While holding them up, perform a clean-type movement to get the dumbbells above your shoulders, but don't attempt to dip under the weight. Instead, use your side and rear delts and traps to move the weight. Don't pause the weight in the top or bottom; just keep it moving up and down in a pumping motion. Rest 2–3 minutes between sets.

BAND PULL-APARTS: Perform 4 sets of 25 reps. Focus on using the rear delts and try to engage the traps as little as possible. Rest 1–2 minutes between sets.

DUMBBELL SHRUGS: Do 2–3 warm-up sets and then perform 4 sets of 25 reps with heavy dumbbells. Use straps so that your grip isn't the limiting factor and just shrug the weight straight up and down with the greatest range of motion possible.

DAY FOUR: ARMS

DOWN-THE-RACK BARBELL CURLS: Warm up then start with a weight that you can get 10 reps with but still have 2–3 reps in the tank. As soon as you get to 10, either strip some weight (loading all 10-pound or 5-pound plates on barbell works well) or grab a barbell that is approximately 10–20% lighter and do another 10 reps. Then do three more drops, performing 10 reps at each drop for a total of 4 drops, which equals 5 sets for a total of 50 reps. Your arms should be totally filled with blood from just one long drop set of this.

STRAIGHT-BAR PUSHDOWN DROP SET: Using the same method as above, warm up and then complete a set of 10 reps with a weight that, at most, would allow you to do 12–13 reps. Then immediately move the pin up a couple holes and do 10 more reps. Keep doing this for a total of 5 drop sets, equaling 50 total reps.

CABLE CURLS: Use a curl-bar attachment on the low pulley. Use a weight that you can get about 20 reps with but only do 15 reps. Do this for 5 sets. The kicker is that you'll only be resting for 45 seconds between sets. Your arms will swell huge from the high volume and short rest periods.

LYING EXTENSIONS WITH CHAINS: Lie flat on your back and perform a skull-crusher-type movement with chains. These can be clipped to D handles or the grenade handles from Elitefts if you have them. Perform 5 sets of 10 reps with only 45 seconds' rest between sets.

REVERSE CURLS WITH EZ-CURL BAR: Use a weight that you can get about 20 reps with but only do 15 reps. Do this for 5 sets. Again, the kicker is that you'll only be resting for 45 seconds between sets. Your biceps and forearms will swell huge from the high volume and short rest periods.

OVERHEAD CABLE EXTENSIONS: Use a rope handle attached to the high pulley. Face away from the machine and bend over at the waist. Extend the rope from behind your head straight out in front of you to arm's length. Perform 5 sets of 10 reps with only 45 seconds' rest between sets.

DAY FIVE: LEGS

CHAIN SQUATS: Warm up by adding only chains to the bar. Once you reach 200 pounds of chains, begin adding plates as you perform 8 reps per set. Keep adding weight until you can no longer get 8 reps. This should take 3–5 work sets. Rest 2–3 minutes between sets.

LEG PRESS: Do 2–3 sets, working up to a weight that requires you to really work to get 20 reps. You are only going to do one all-out work set here, but the trick is that you are going to find a way to get 40 reps with a weight that would be difficult to get 20 with. Pause at lockout, push with your hands on your knees—do whatever you have to do to get all 40 reps in one set without racking the weight. Really push yourself here and resist the temptation to wimp out and take a weight you know you can do.

CHAIN LUNGES: Throw the appropriate amount of chains around your neck and take 30 steps (15 reps with each leg), touching your knee to the ground on each step. Do this for 4 sets of 30 steps. Rest 2–3 minutes between sets.

BARBELL STIFF-LEGGED DEADS: Use 25-pound plates for these or stand on a 4-inch platform to increase the range of motion. Keep your chest up and lower back arched and concentrate on using your hams to move the weight. Keep a slight bend in your knees throughout the movement. Do not rest the weight on the floor during the set; keep tension on the muscles at all times. Work up to a hard set of 10 reps and then stay there for 4 sets of 10 reps. Rest 2–3 minutes between sets.

LYING LEG CURLS: After one or two feeder sets, perform 4 sets of 25 reps. If you don't have a machine, use bands while sitting on a bench with the bands attached to a sturdy structure about 3–4 feet away. Rest 2–3 minutes between sets.

CALF TRISET: After warming up a bit, start with calf raises on the leg-press machine and use a weight that allows 20 reps. Get off the leg press and immediately start doing standing calf raises off an elevated platform with just your body weight for 25 reps. Then go immediately to the seated calf machine and do another 20 reps. Repeat this three times, and you're done for the day. Rest 2–3 minutes between sets.

WEEK TEN

DAY ONE: CHEST

INCLINE DUMBBELL PRESSES: Use a low incline that is only at an angle of approximately 15–25 degrees. In 2–3 sets, work up to a fairly tough set of 10 reps and stay there for 4 sets of 10 reps. Rest 2–3 minutes between sets.

STANDARD BENCH PRESS: After a warm-up set or two, take a weight at or close to your 5-rep max. Then perform 5 sets of 5 reps, but decrease the weight on the bar by 10 pounds each set. If your 5-rep max was 400 × 5, your session would look like this: 400 × 5, 390 × 5, 380 × 5, 370 × 5, 360 × 5. Rest 2–3 minutes between sets.

DUMBBELL TWIST PRESSES: Perform these by starting just as you would for a traditional dumbbell bench press. As you press the weight up, however, twist your wrists so that, at the top of the movement, your palms are supinated like a reverse-grip bench press. Then touch the ends of the dumbbells together. Start light and work up in small increments for sets of 10 reps until you can no longer fully rotate the dumbbells at the top. This is much harder than a regular dumbbell bench press. I want at least 4 of these sets to be work sets. Rest 2–3 minutes between sets.

DAY TWO: BACK

ONE-ARM BARBELL ROWS: If you have a Meadows row handle, use it for these. If not, just grasp the barbell at the very end near the inside collar. Place the other end of the barbell in a landmine apparatus or shove it into a corner. Load just the one end of the barbell and use 25-pound or 10-pound plates on these to allow for a full range of motion. Work up to a max set of 10 reps. Work hard and set a PR here. At least 3–4 sets should be work sets. Rest 2–3 minutes between sets.

LAT PULL-DOWNS WITH AN UNDERHAND GRIP: Use a standard, wide, straight pull-down bar attachment for lats that allows you to take a wide grip, but take an underhand grip as if you were going to perform curls on it. Try to take the biceps out of the movement as much as possible and focus on using your lats throughout the movement by pulling from your elbows. After two feeder sets, pick a weight that will require you to work hard to get 10 reps, then stay there for 4 sets of 10 reps. Rest 2–3 minutes between sets.

T-BAR ROWS: Use a V handle with a barbell in a landmine-type device or with the end of the barbell shoved in a corner. Work up a 45 pound plate (or 25-pound plate at a time depending on your strength level) at 10 reps per set until you can no longer get 10 reps. At least 4 of these should be work sets. Rest 2–3 minutes between sets.

BARBELL SHRUGS: Use a double overhand and just focus on moving your shoulders up and down (after warming up) with as much weight as possible for 3 sets of 20 reps.

HYPEREXTENSIONS WITH A LIGHT BAND: Use a light band and do one all-out, balls-to-the-wall set to failure. Push yourself on these, get a PR, and then you're done for the day.

DAY THREE: SHOULDERS

LEANING LATERAL RAISES: Grab onto a sturdy structure with one hand and hold the dumbbell in the other. Keeping your feet together and close to the structure, lean away from it until your arm is straight. This will make the movement very strict and hit the medial delt hard. After 1–2 warm-ups, perform 3 sets of 20 reps with a smooth and controlled tempo. Rest 2–3 minutes between sets.

SEATED DUMBBELL PRESSES: Work up slowly in sets of 8 reps until you reach your max set of 8. At least 4 of these should feel like work sets. Rest 2–3 minutes between sets.

SEATED BENT LATERAL RAISES: Perform 3 sets of 20 reps. Focus on using the rear delts and try to engage the traps as little as possible. Rest 2–3 minutes between sets.

BARBELL SHRUGS: Perform 2–3 feeder sets and then do 5 sets of 10 reps, as heavy as possible. Just shrug the weight straight up and down since there is no reason to roll your shoulders or move them in a horizontal plane during the movement.

DAY FOUR: ARMS

STRAIGHT-BAR CURLS: Warm up, then start with a weight that you can get 10 reps with but still have 4–5 reps in the tank. Do this for 5 sets. The kicker is that you'll only be resting for 45 seconds between sets for every exercise today and doing 5 sets of 10 reps on everything. Your arms will swell huge from the high volume and short rest periods.

ROPE PUSHDOWNS: Warm up, then start with a weight that you can get 10 reps with but still have 4–5 reps in the tank. Then perform 5 sets of 10 reps with 45 seconds' rest between sets.

DUMBBELL HAMMER CURLS: Keep your elbows at your sides and, again, do all the reps with both arms at the same time. Perform 5 sets of 10 reps with 45 seconds' rest between sets.

SKULL CRUSHERS WITH CHAINS: Lie flat on your back and perform a skull-crusher-type movement with chains using an EZ-curl bar. Again, use a weight that would normally allow you to get at least 15 reps for one set. Perform 5 sets of 10 reps with only 45 seconds' rest between sets.

CABLE CURLS: Use a curl-bar attachment on the low pulley. Again, use a weight that would normally allow you to get at least 15 reps for one set. Perform 5 sets of 10 reps with only 45 seconds' rest between sets.

BENCH DIPS: Body weight is all you should need by the time you get here, but if you're feeling good, add weight by placing plates in your lap. Set up two benches of the same height. Perform dips in between them, keeping your legs straight, your feet on one bench, and your hands on the bench just behind you. Perform 5 sets of 10 reps with only 45 seconds rest between sets.

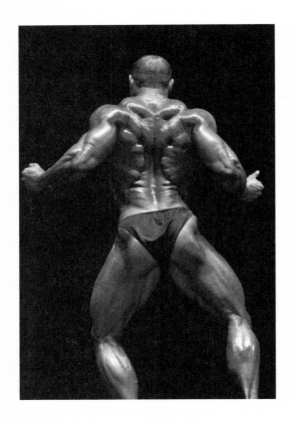

DAY FIVE: LEGS

REVERSE BAND SQUATS: Use medium or heavy bands suspended from the top of the squat rack for these. Warm up and then work up to a max set of 10 reps. And by "max," I mean that I want you to get the heaviest set of 10 reps that you can. This should take 3–5 work sets, not counting warm-up sets. Rest 2–4 minutes between sets.

LEG PRESS: Today you are going to do a monster of a drop set. After 1–2 feeder sets, pick a weight that is as close to a true 10-rep max as possible, but only load the leg-press machine with 45-pound plates. You are only going to do one set, but make it count. Do your set of 10 reps and, without racking the weight, have your training partners strip a plate; perform 10 more reps. Do this one plate per side per set until there are no longer any plates left on the machine. If you're fairly strong, this could be as many as ten sets or more. Dig down and don't stop until there aren't any plates left.

BULGARIAN SPLIT SQUATS: Put one foot up on a bench behind you with the other foot out front. Squat down on your front leg so that you're in a lunge-type position in the bottom and then push back up with your front leg. If these squats are too easy with just body weight, add resistance by placing chains around your neck. After the first two movements, however, I seriously doubt that the squats will be too easy. Perform 4 sets of 15 reps with each leg. Rest 2–3 minutes between sets.

DUMBBELL STIFF-LEGGED DEADS: Keep your chest up and lower back arched and concentrate on using your hams to move the weight.

Keep a slight bend in your knees throughout the movement. Do not rest the weight on the floor during the set; keep tension on the muscles at all times. Work up to a hard set of 10 reps and then stay there for 4 sets of 10 reps. Rest 2–3 minutes between sets.

SEATED LEG CURLS: Work up to a fairly tough set of 10 reps. For your next set, keep the weight the same but perform 15 reps. For your third set, again keep the weight the same but find a way to get 20 reps. If you fail, have your partner assist you with forced reps until you hit the desired number. If you don't have a machine, use bands while sitting on a bench with the bands attached to a sturdy structure about 3–4 feet away. Rest 2–3 minutes between sets.

STANDING CALF RAISES: Warm up well, then do 4 sets of 25 reps.

SEATED CALF RAISES: Perform 4 sets of 25 reps.

DONKEY CALF RAISES: You can perform these on a machine if your gym has one. Or, have a training partner (or two) sit on your back while placing your toes on a four-by-four-inch block or something similar to increase your range of motion. With partners is how Arnold performed these back in the '70s. Again, do 4 sets of 25 reps.

WEEK ELEVEN

DAY ONE: CHEST

CHAIN BENCH PRESS: Use approximately 100 pounds in chains and then add plates before each set to increase the weight. Warm up and work up to a max set of 6 reps. Work hard and try to set a new PR here. This should take 3–5 work sets, not counting warm-up sets. Rest 2–4 minutes between sets.

INCLINE BARBELL PRESSES: Use a low incline that is only at an angle of approximately 15–25 degrees. After a warm-up set or two, take a weight at or close to your 5-rep max. Then perform 5 sets of 10 reps but decrease the weight on the bar by 10 pounds each set. If your 10-rep max was 315 × 10, your session would look like this: 315 × 10, 305 × 10, 295 × 10, 285 × 10, 275 × 10. Rest 2–3 minutes between sets.

CHAIN FLIES: Clip D handles to chains and, after 1–2 warm-ups, perform 4 sets of 15 reps with a smooth and controlled tempo. At the top of the rep, touch the handles together while supinating your hands so that your pinkies touch. This will elicit a very full contraction.

LADDER PUSH-UPS: You can put a bar inside a power cage for these, setting pins at three different heights. Or, use a Smith machine if you have access to one. The first setting should be as low to the ground as possible. Pump out as many reps as possible but stop 2–4 reps short of complete failure. Move the bar up six to ten inches and pump out as many as possible, this time going to failure. Then move the bar up another six to ten inches and go again until failure. Your chest should be totally engorged with blood at this point. If you can do more than 25 reps on the first set, add resistance by having your training partners drape chains across your back in an X. Perform just one all-out set and go until you have nothing left.

DAY TWO: BACK

KROC ROWS: Do 2–3 warm-up sets, then 1 × 40 (yes, 40 reps); go as heavy as possible on these but don't use straps. Try to beat whatever your PR is or set a new one. It is only necessary to do one set for each arm, but be sure to take a weight here that really challenges you.

NEUTRAL-GRIP LAT PULL-DOWNS: Use a bar that allows you to take a medium-to-wide, neutral grip. Try to take the biceps out of the movement as much as possible and focus on using your lats throughout the movement by pulling from your elbows. After two feeder sets, pick a weight that will require you to work hard to get 10 reps, then stay there for 4 sets of 10 reps. Rest 2–3 minutes between sets.

CHEST-SUPPORTED ROWS: Pyramid up in weight for sets of 15, 12, 10, 8. Rest 2–3 minutes between sets.

DUMBBELL PULLOVERS: Keep your arms straight (or maintain a slight bend in the elbows) and concentrate on using your lats, really flexing them hard at the top. Avoid using a really long range of motion, which turns the pullover into a triceps movement. Just go back until you feel a full stretch in your lats, not allowing your arms to bend, and bring the dumbbell at the top over your chin/neck area. You'll find that your reps will get slightly deeper as the set progresses. Perform 4 sets of 10 reps.

DUMBBELL SHRUGS: Use straps and hold each rep at the top for 2 seconds with the traps fully contracted. Perform 3 sets of 10 reps. Rest 2–3 minutes between sets.

DAY THREE: SHOULDERS

SEATED CHAIN LATERAL RAISES: Clip D handles to chains and, after 1–2 warm-ups, perform 3 sets of 20 reps with a smooth and controlled tempo. On the last rep, hold the weight at lockout for as long as possible. Concentrate on using your medial delts to move the weight and avoid shrugging your shoulders up or back to keep the traps out of the movement as much as possible. Rest 2–3 minutes between sets.

BAND PULL-APARTS: Perform 4 sets of 25 reps. Focus on using the rear delts and try to engage the traps as little as possible. Rest 1–2 minutes between sets.

STANDING MILITARY PRESSES: Another reverse pyramid here. Work up in 2–3 sets to a tough set of 5 reps. Decrease the weight by 10–15% and do a set of 10 reps. Then decrease the weight by 10–15% and do a set of 15 reps. Then decrease the weight by 10–15% and do a set of 20 reps. Rest 2–3 minutes between sets.

DUMBBELL SHRUGS: Do 2–3 warm-up sets and then perform 4 sets of 25 reps with heavy dumbbells. Use straps here so that your grip isn't the limiting factor and just shrug the weight straight up and down with the greatest range of motion possible.

DAY FOUR: ARMS

DOWN-THE-RACK BARBELL CURLS: Warm up, then start with a weight that you can get 10 reps with but still have 2–3 reps in the tank. As soon as you get to 10, either strip some weight (loading all 10-pound or 5-pound plates on the barbell works well) or grab a barbell that is approximately 10-20% lighter and do another 10 reps. Then drop again and do 10 reps at each drop for a total of 4 drops, which equals 5 sets for a total of 50 reps. Your arms should be totally filled with blood from just one long drop set of this.

DUMBBELL CURLS: Keep your palm supinated at all times (palm up) and perform all reps with one arm, then switch to the other arm. Perform 10 reps per set.

SUPERSETTED WITH:

DUMBBELL HAMMER CURLS: Do these straight up and down like a regular curl, not across the body. Again, perform all reps with one arm, then switch to the other arm. Perform 10 reps per set.

Perform 4 sets of each superset for 8 sets total between the two exercises. Rest 2–3 minutes between each superset.

EZ-BAR PREACHER REVERSE CURLS: Perform 10 reps per set. Start this superset with your palms facing down in a reverse-curl fashion.

SUPERSETTED WITH:

EZ-BAR PREACHER CURLS: Just reverse your grip so that your palms face up and keep going. Perform 10 reps per set.

Perform 4 sets of each superset for 8 sets total between the two exercises. Rest 2–3 minutes between each superset.

ROPE PUSHDOWNS: Get full extension and push the rope apart at the bottom. Perform 15 reps per set.

SUPERSETTED WITH:

OVERHEAD ROPE EXTENSIONS: Simply turn around after finishing the pushdowns and do another 15 reps, but lean away from the machine and extend the rope overhead. It is okay to lighten the weight some if necessary to complete all the reps.

Perform 4 sets of each superset for 8 sets total between the two exercises. Rest 2–3 minutes between each super set.

OVERHEAD DUMBBELL EXTENSIONS: Get full extension at the top and a decent stretch at the bottom. Perform 15 reps per set.

SUPERSETTED WITH:

BENCH DIPS: Set up two benches of the same height and perform dips in between them. Have your partner place plates in your lap to add resistance. Perform 20 reps per set.

Perform 4 sets of each superset for 8 sets total between the two exercises. Rest 2–3 minutes between each superset.

SKULL-CRUSHER DROP SET: Your elbows should be warmed up well by now, so do one warm-up set and then start with a weight that you can get 12–15 reps with but only do 10. As soon as you get to 10, strip some weight (loading all 10-pound or 5-pound plates on barbell works well)—approximately 10–20%—and do another 10 reps. Then drop again and do 10 reps at each drop for a total of 4 drops, which equals 5 sets for a total of 50 reps. Your arms should be totally filled with blood from just one long drop set of this.

DAY FIVE: LEGS

SQUATS: These are regular old back squats, but what you will do isn't normal at all. Warm up in 3–4 sets and then pick a weight that requires you to strain to get 10–12 reps. You are going to do one long and difficult drop set consisting of 4 drops (after your initial set) of 8 reps each (for a total of 5 sets and 40 reps, all in one single prolonged set). The bar should only be racked long enough to have your partners strip the plates, and the weight should be reduced approximately 15–20% on each drop. Keep a bucket near for this one.

LEG PRESS: Perform just 1–2 feeder sets and then do 4 sets of 10 reps with a weight that has you struggling by the last set. Rest 2–3 minutes between sets.

CHAIN LUNGES: Throw the appropriate amount of chains around your neck and take 30 steps (15 reps with each leg), touching your knee to the ground on each step. Do this for 3 sets of 30 steps. Rest 2–3 minutes between sets.

BARBELL STIFF-LEGGED DEADS: Use 25-pound plates for these or stand on a four-inch platform to increase the range of motion. Keep your chest up and lower back arched and concentrate on using your hams to move the weight. Keep a slight bend in your knees throughout the movement. Do not rest the weight on the floor during the set; keep tension on the muscles at all times. Work up to a hard set of 15 reps and then stay there for 3 sets of 15 reps. Rest 2–3 minutes between sets.

LYING LEG CURLS: After one to two feeder sets, perform 4 sets of 25 reps. If you don't have a machine, use bands while sitting on a bench with the bands attached to a sturdy structure about 3–4 feet away. Rest 2–3 minutes between sets.

CALF TRISET: After warming up a bit, start with calf raises on the leg-press machine and use a weight that allows 20 reps. Get off the leg press and immediately start doing standing calf raises off an elevated platform with just your body weight for 25 reps. Then go immediately to the seated calf machine and do another 20 reps. Repeat this three times, and you're done for the day. Rest 2–3 minutes between sets.

WEEK TWELVE

DAY ONE: CHEST

DECLINE DUMBBELL PRESS: Warm up well and then work up slowly to an 8-rep max, making at least four of the sets work sets.

INCLINE BARBELL PRESS: Perform 2–3 warm-up sets and then work up slowly to an 8-rep max, making at least four of the sets work sets.

BANDED BENCH PRESS: Use long red pro minibands for these and set it up so that the bands are pulling down against you. Pick a moderate weight and do 8 sets of 3 reps, attempting to move the bar on the concentric phase as fast as possible. Only take 60-second rest periods between sets.

DUMBBELL OR CHAIN FLIES: Do 3 sets of 20.

DAY TWO: BACK

DEAD-STOP BARBELL ROW: Perform these inside a power rack and set pins at mid shin height. At the bottom of each rep pause the weight briefly on the pins. Do 2–3 warm-up sets and then do 4 sets of 10, adding weight each set.

UNDERHAND GRIP PULL-DOWNS: These will focus on your lower lats. Do 4 sets of 8 here. Really focus on contracting and squeezing your lower lats on the way down.

DEADLIFTS: Use conventional deadlift form and work up slowly to a 5-rep max.

RACK PULLS: Set the pins so the bar is resting just below your knees at the start. Work up to a heavy triple.

DUMBBELL PULLOVERS: Perform 3 sets of 12. Remember to focus on only using your lats to move the weight.

HYPEREXTENSIONS: Do 1 set to complete failure with body weight only. Shoot for 50 reps.

DAY THREE: SHOULDERS

SEATED DUMBBELL POWER CLEANS: Do 3 sets of 25 reps with 60-second rest periods.

PLATE RAISES: Perform 5 sets of 10 reps with 30-second rest periods.

BAND PULL-APARTS: Do 5 sets of 10 reps with 30-second rest periods.

BARBELL SHRUGS: Perform 2–3 feeder sets and then do 5 sets of 10 reps, as heavy as possible. Just shrug the weight straight up and down since there is no reason to roll your shoulders or move them in a horizontal plane during the movement.

DAY FOUR: BICEPS/TRICEPS

SEATED BARBELL CURL: Perform several warm-up sets and then pick a weight that is challenging for 5 sets of 10 reps, resting 60 seconds between sets.

HAMMER CURL: Do 3 sets of 10 here with a full range of motion, plus 6 partial reps out of the bottom on all 3 sets.

CABLE CURL: Do these with the 21 technique. The first 7 reps are the bottom half only, the next 7 reps are top half only, and the last 7 are full range of motion. Perform 3 sets of 21 reps.

PREACHER CURLS: Do 3 sets of 15 with 30-second breaks.

ROPE PUSHDOWNS: Keep your hands in close to your body and push your elbows out. Flex at the bottom for 1 second. Do 3 sets of 20.

DIP MACHINE OR BENCH DIPS: Use a dip machine (or do bench dips with weight in your lap) for 3 sets of 15. Lower yourself slowly and focus on using your triceps.

INCLINE LYING EXTENSION: On these, do 3 sets of 12 with good form.

SEATED OVERHEAD ROPE EXTENSIONS: For this, you are seated with a back support facing away from the cable machine. Do 5 sets of 15 with 30-second breaks.

DAY FIVE: LEGS

LEG PRESS: Do sets of 20 reps, adding one plate per side on each set until you can no longer get 20 reps. Rest 2–3 minutes between sets.

BARBELL SQUATS: Do one to two feeder sets, then do 4 sets of 15 with a challenging weight.

WALKING LUNGES: Do these one leg at a time. This means you lunge down and then bring the trail leg back to where feet are even. Then you lunge again with the same leg until all of the reps are completed with one leg. Without rest, immediately perform all the reps with the opposite leg. Add weight with chains or a barbell across your shoulders. Perform 3 sets of 15 reps with each leg.

BARBELL STIFF-LEGGED DEADLIFT: Use 25-pound plates to allow for a better stretch. Keep the bar in nice and tight against your body and push your hips back as you descend. Work up in sets of 8 reps, starting with just the bar and adding a 25-pound plate to each side at every set until you can no longer achieve 8 reps in good form.

LYING LEG CURLS: Do 4 sets of 15 with 30-second breaks.

STANDING CALF RAISES: Warm up well, then do 4 sets of 25 reps.

SEATED CALF RAISES: Perform 4 sets of 25 reps.

DONKEY CALF RAISES: You can perform these on a machine if your gym has one. Or, have a training partner (or two) sit on your back while placing your toes on a four-by-four-inch block or something similar to increase your range of motion. With partners is how Arnold performed these back in the '70s. Again, do 4 sets of 25 reps.

FIFTEEN
NUTRITION

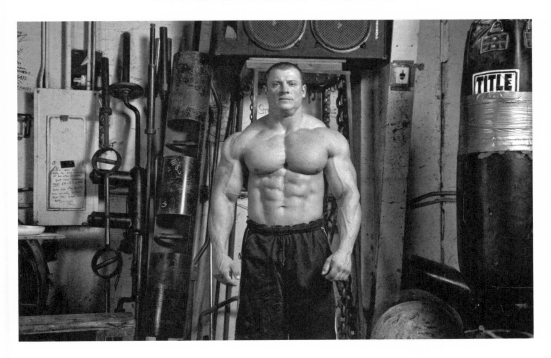

Although this is a book about training, since diet plays such a substantial role in the success of our training, it would be remiss not to at least touch on it. I'm not going to go into a lot of detail since that would be another book in itself, but I do want to at least provide you with some good diet basics to get you on the right path and to help you put the right fuel in your machine.

WEIGHT LOSS/GAIN VERSUS BODY COMPOSITION

It is basic physics and undeniable that to lose weight, people must consume fewer calories than they burn and that to gain weight, caloric intake must exceed expenditure. By accepting this simple rule, we recognize that it is the amount of food that will cause either weight loss or gain. However, that oversimplifies things and does not give us a good view of the overall picture. While the amount of food may determine if we are losing or gaining weight, it is the quality of those calories that will play a large role in determining how our body composition is affected. Two diets comprised of the same number of calories may both elicit the same change in body weight, but it is the quality of food, ratio of macronutrients, and timing of the intake of those nutrients that will play a major role in how much fat is lost or how much muscle is gained.

MACRONUTRIENTS

CARBOHYDRATES

While the optimal ratio of fats to protein to carbohydrates will vary greatly depending on your body composition, metabolism, activity level, and goals, I do believe that there are basics that apply to the majority of athletes. That being said, there are exceptions to every rule, and diets should always be tailored to the specific needs of the individual athlete. Generally speaking, the macronutrient that will be manipulated or altered the most depending on whether an individual is attempting to diet off adipose tissue or induce muscular hypertrophy will be carbohydrates. Carbohydrate intake will typically be reduced when attempting to lose body fat and increased when attempting to gain new muscle mass. Carbohydrate intake can also vary greatly between individuals with similar goals but possessing different metabolisms and body composition. Typically, individuals who tend to gain weight and body fat easily (classic endomorphs) will perform better on diets comprised of fewer carbs than individuals who have a hard time gaining weight but are naturally lean (classic ectomorphs), who usually require a higher carbohydrate intake.

PROTEIN

I am a proponent of a relatively high protein intake for athletes looking to gain muscle or those in a dieting phase who are attempting to reduce body fat while retaining as much muscle mass as possible. For the majority of hard-training athletes, I recommend one gram of protein per pound of body weight, and for extremely muscular hard-training individuals (think professional powerlifters and bodybuilders), as much as two grams per pound of body weight may be optimal. You may have heard the claim that high-protein intake is bad for your kidneys, but this contention requires further examination. While there is evidence that a high-protein intake can be harmful to an individual with preexisting kidney damage, to my knowledge no study has shown that a high-protein diet in healthy individuals causes kidney problems. You will want to make the majority of protein selections from low-fat sources like chicken breasts, turkey breasts, white fish, egg whites, and lean cuts of red meat. Furthermore, I recommend trimming away any visible fat before cooking to eliminate as much saturated fat as possible.

FATS

I also believe consuming a sufficient amount of healthy fats is very important not only to an individual's overall health but also to his or her performance. While there is some degree of dissension among nutrition experts about exactly which fats are bad or good, there is definitely some consensus. Fats high in omega-3 (polyunsaturated fats) and omega-9 (monounsaturated fats) are generally considered beneficial when consumed in moderation. Coconut oil, while technically a saturated fat, is a specific type called a medium-chain triglyceride and processed differently by the body than other saturated fats. Some research has shown that consuming coconut oil can aid in increasing HDL cholesterol levels (the good cholesterol). One thing the experts universally agree on is that trans fats are to be avoided as much as possible. These are fats that are partially hydrogenated, and, while some occur naturally, the majority are produced artificially and found in abundance in highly processed food.

VEGETABLES

Vegetables can range from being high in vitamins and minerals to being comprised principally of roughage. However, most provide a low caloric load and are great "fillers" on a diet, when hunger is a frequent adversary.

CONDIMENTS, SPICES, AND BEVERAGES

Any zero-calorie condiments can be used liberally. Many bodybuilders are big fans of mustard and low-carb hot sauces, which add flavor and increase palatability. Almost any spice can be used to make food more flavorful since they typically do not contain any calories. Any beverage that is zero-calorie (diet soda, black coffee, unsweetened tea, Crystal Light, etc.) can be consumed without having a negative effect on the athlete's diet, but if overall health is a primary concern, plain old drinking water is likely best.

The following lists, by no means exhaustive, provide some options for each of the different categories of food.

PROTEIN:

chicken, lean cuts of steak, white fish, turkey, egg whites, any high-quality whey- or casein-based protein powders

CARBOHYDRATES:

rice (brown, white, basmati, etc.), potatoes, yams or sweet potatoes, oatmeal, Cream of Rice, Malt-O-Meal, Ezekiel bread

FATS:

FRUITS: avocados, olives, coconut oil
NUTS: almonds, pistachios, walnuts
OILS: canola, olive and sunflower
COLD-WATER FISH: herring, mackerel, salmon, trout, tuna

VEGETABLES:

salad greens, broccoli, cauliflower, asparagus, spinach, green beans

PERI-TRAINING NUTRITION

Peri-training nutrition is something that has received more attention recently and deservedly so. It consists of what an athlete consumes before, during, and immediately following training. There is strong evidence suggesting that properly structuring what an athlete eats during this time frame can have a significant impact on post-training recovery and fueling muscles during training. It can also inhibit muscle breakdown due to training and thus significantly reduce or eliminate delayed-onset muscle soreness (DOMS).

PRETRAINING

Approximately one hour before training, a combination of complex carbs, fat-free protein, and a small amount of healthy fats should be consumed. The carbs will provide fuel for the muscles, the protein aids in repair and hypertrophy, and the fat is there to provide a slow, even release of the nutrients by slow gastric emptying. An example for a hard-training adult male would be fifty grams of whey isolate, half a cup of oatmeal, and one tablespoon of all-natural peanut butter one hour before training.

INTRAWORKOUT

During the actual training session, it is imperative to continue feeding the athlete's muscles. Here you want fast-absorbing and easily digestible protein and carbohydrate sources in a one-to-three ratio. This should be in a form that can be dissolved in water to be sipped during training. The nutrients need to get into the bloodstream quickly and should not cause a full feeling or gastric distress. Hydrolyzed casein and highly branched cyclic dextrin are the preferred sources since they exist in a form that our body can use with minimum digestion. However, they can be expensive, and hydrolyzed casein may require strong flavoring to mask the bitterness. It can be purchased in a form that is not bitter, but this further increases the cost of what is already a fairly expensive supplement (at least as of the publishing of this book). A cheaper alternative is whey-isolate protein powder mixed in Gatorade (sucrose). While this does require some digestion and doesn't provide all the benefits of hydrolyzed casein combined with cyclic dextrin, it is still absorbed relatively quickly, is quite palatable, and is much less expensive. I have found that vanilla-flavored whey-isolate tastes pleasant when mixed with fruit punch or orange-flavored Gatorade. An example for a lean 200–pound athlete would be thirty grams of hydrolyzed casein combined with ninety grams of cyclic dextrin and dissolved in fifty ounces of water or thirty grams of whey isolate mixed in fifty ounces of Gatorade.

POST-TRAINING

Approximately one hour after training (or sooner if possible), the post-training meal should be consumed. It would ideally consist of a lean protein source (chicken, white fish, or very lean red meat) and a clean, very low-fat carbohydrate source (I prefer white rice). Fat should be avoided as much as possible at this meal because it will slow gastric emptying and delay the delivery of the nutrients to the muscles.

SIXTEEN
TOP TEN THINGS YOU MUST DO TO GET INSANELY STRONG

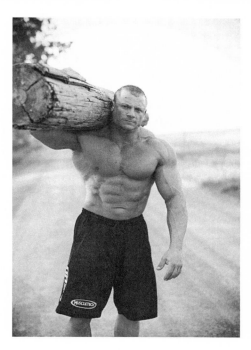

1. Constantly strive for progress in your training (can be in amount of weight lifted, reps, or volume).
2. You must eat like it is your job. You must consume the right food and enough of it to reach your goals. The further you progress, the more important this becomes.
3. You must be willing to train through pain and discomfort. Heavy lifting requires mental strength as much as it does physical.

173

4. You must be willing to train around and through injuries. The stronger you get and the heavier the weights are that you handle, the more likely you are to become injured. The guys at the top accept this as part of the process of becoming one of the strongest. It isn't whether you get injured but, rather, how you deal with it when you do that ultimately determines how far you will go.

5. You must be willing to do what others are not. In order to separate yourself from the crowd, you must push yourself to places others cannot go.

6. You must realize that numbers mean nothing. You cannot let a certain number intimidate you in any lift. Recognize that many others have lifted more weight than you and that it can be done. No weight is impossible to lift, even a weight that no one has ever lifted.

7. Learn to focus on the numbers that are just ahead of your current capabilities, and the distant ones will soon be closer.

8. You must be passionate about wanting to be stronger. Getting ridiculously strong requires working extremely hard for years and enduring vast amounts of pain. If you don't go to bed thinking about getting stronger, wake up thinking about getting stronger, and think about getting stronger all throughout the day, then you may want to pursue a different endeavor.

9. You must realize that there are no reasons for not getting stronger, only excuses. Injuries, your career (or lack thereof), lack of money, poor genetics, no time, etcetera are all excuses. Accept this and you'll instantly be much closer to accomplishing your goals.

10. You must be at least a little insane.

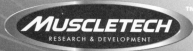

THE MOST POWERFUL SUPPLEMENTS ON EARTH.™

BECOME A MASS MONSTER

MASS TECH

MUSCLETECH
PERFORMANCE SERIES

7 lbs
NEW SIZE
MORE SERVINGS

ADVANCED MUSCLE MASS GAINER

DESIGNED FOR THE HARDGAINER
BUILD MASS & STRENGTH
MULTI-PHASE PROTEIN SYSTEM
FORMULATED WITH OMEGA-9 COMPOUNDS

MILK CHOCOLATE
NATURAL AND ARTIFICIAL FLAVORS

MATT KROCZALESKI
WORLD CHAMPION POWERLIFTER
@MattKroc

🐦 f 🔵 **MUSCLETECH**.COM

MASS-TECH® is the world's most advanced mass gainer engineered to deliver 80g of quality protein to fuel your quest for monstrous muscle gains. Powerfully formulated to supply your high-octane metabolism with a massive 1,170 calories and a clinically validated dose of 10g of creatine, MASS-TECH® is the hard-gainer's solution for superior size and strength.

80g Protein‡
Delivers 80g of quality protein – that's more than other big-name gainers out there! It also supplies fast-, medium-, and slow-digesting proteins, providing amino acids to the body at varying speeds for extended delivery

1170 Calories‡
Delivers a massive 1,170 calories from high-quality protein, quickly digested carbohydrates, and specialized fats. It's the most versatile weight gainer available, and can be taken in two separate half servings throughout the day

13g BCAAs‡
Supplies a massive 13g of BCAAs and 7g of leucine, which help fuel your skeletal muscles, preserve muscle glycogen stores, and help reduce the amount of protein breakdown

10g Creatine
MASS-TECH® delivers a 10g clinically validated dose to increase strength fast, unlike other gainers

‡When mixed with 2 cups of skim milk. Facebook logo is owned by Facebook Inc. Read the entire label and follow directions. © 2014